Teen Parenting

Look for these and other books in the Lucent
Overview Series:

Teen Parenting

by Gail B. Stewart

TEEN ISSUES

LUCENT *Overview Series*

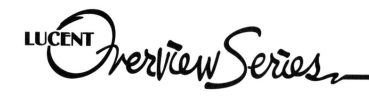

Library of Congress Cataloging-in-Publication Data

Stewart, Gail B., 1949–
    Teen Parenting / by Gail B. Stewart.
        p.   cm. — (Teen issues)
    Includes bibliographical references and index.
    Summary: Discusses life as a teenage parent, the cost to society, future goals of public policy on the topic, alternatives to becoming a teenage parent, and the programs to help teens make the transition to parenthood.
    ISBN 1-56006-517-6
    1. Teenage parents—United States Juvenile literature. 2. Teenage pregnancy— United States Juvenile literature. 3. Teenage parents—Government policy—United States Juvenile literature. [1. Teenage parents. 2. Pregnancy.] I. Title. II. Series.
HQ759.64.M39   2000
306.874'3—dc21
                                              99-37624
                                                CIP

Copyright © 2000 by Lucent Books, Inc.
P.O. Box 289011, San Diego, CA 92198-9011
Printed in the U.S.A.

Contents

Introduction

IN A SUBURB north of Minneapolis, eighteen-year-old Mary sits on a sofa holding her infant daughter, who's teething. Having been up with her daughter most of the previous night, Mary is pale and weary-looking. Her boyfriend, Jamie, is downstairs in the basement with friends, and the high-pitched beeps indicate that a Nintendo game is in progress. "That's sort of what Jamie does, is play Nintendo," she says, shifting the baby to her other shoulder. "I love being with my baby, but I really wish he'd help out more."[1]

"Six kids, with five different fathers"

Trina, another young mother, is sitting on a patch of grass near a homeless shelter smoking a cigarette. Five of her children stand aimlessly nearby, unsure of what to do with themselves. Her sixth child, a newborn, dozes in her arms.

"Six kids, with five different fathers," she says quietly. "That's gotta be some kind of record, huh? I can't say it was a mistake, because that would be disrespecting my children. It would be like saying they shouldn't be here. But I will say that most of those babies' fathers were mistakes. I got into some things I'd have been better off leaving alone—especially crack."

Trina shrugs when asked what being a mother is like.

"I'm a recovering addict, four days ago I delivered my sixth child, and we're homeless. I guess right now it seems like things couldn't get no worse."[2]

"Mostly, I'm sad"

Although she would rank her life above Trina's right now, nineteen-year-old Kay is far from happy about her situation. She is in a hurry to get to her high school class, and her daughter is fooling around instead of finding her shoes. Repeated attempts to move the little girl along are falling on deaf ears.

Kay says that although she loves her daughter, she resents the loss of her own childhood. "Mostly, for me, it's that I've lost out on my teenage years," Kay says flatly.

> I get jealous of other people, of how they live, the things they do. I hear girls say, "I'm going to go to college in Florida." I wish I could go to college in Florida. I want to go to a college far away, someplace great like Florida.

A nineteen-year-old single parent talks to her son. It is becoming more and more common to see children with teenage parents.

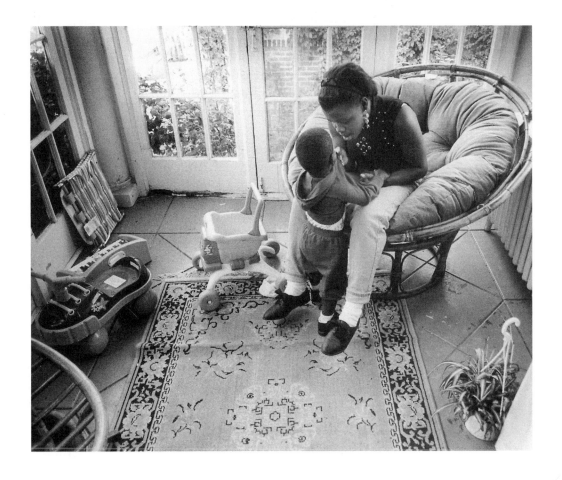

As for my daughter, I like making her happy. It's fun to see her when I tell her we're going somewhere or when I buy her a present that she really likes. But other than that, I'm not glad she's born. Mostly, I'm sad. Every day it goes through my head; I can't stop thinking about it. I feel guilty, too, like I'm supposed to think a different way. I just live with it, though.[3]

A common bond

Mary, Trina, and Kay are very different people, with very different upbringings—yet they share the common bond of becoming parents at a very early age. They are part of a rapidly growing group of teen parents in the United States—more than 500,000 each year. Only a small fraction of teens who give birth—roughly 3 percent—give their babies up for adoption. The rest decide to keep their babies.

Not only are the numbers of teen parents increasing daily, say experts, but the age at which teens are starting families is getting dramatically younger. In fact, in a recent study, researchers Barbara and Richard Lowenthal found that the fastest-growing group of parents in the United States are girls between the ages of ten and fourteen.

Most of the 1 million teenagers who become pregnant each year are unmarried; by far, the majority of pregnancies are unplanned. Unprepared for the physical, financial, and emotional stresses of pregnancy, teen mothers—as well as teen fathers—can easily be overwhelmed.

Bleak consequences

The increase in the numbers of teen parents in the United States has prompted a great deal of concern—from politicians, social workers, and educators. Study after study has been done to monitor teen parents, and to understand the problems that they face.

These studies suggest that one of the most common problems for teen parents is poverty. One 1997 report, *Kids Having Kids: Economic Costs and Social Consequences of Teen Pregnancy,* foretells bleak consequences for teen mothers and their children, claiming that "more than 80 percent end up in poverty and reliant on welfare, many for the majority of their children's critically important developmental years."[4]

In addition, the report finds that children of teen mothers are far more likely to do poorly in school, be abused or neglected, and engage in criminal activity. The cost society bears for these children in terms of welfare, courts, and medical care is astronomical—almost $7 billion per year.

Health risks

One especially worrisome aspect of the issue is the health of babies born to teen mothers. Experts say that teens are more likely to give birth to babies with low birth weight or other health problems. These are often the result of poor prenatal care.

The reason for many teens' poor prenatal care, say doctors, is that they do not see a doctor early in their pregnancy. This is especially true of young teens ages thirteen to fifteen. Because of their age and the understandable ignorance about conception or the physical growth of a fetus, many teens don't realize they are pregnant until the third or fourth month. And by that time, they might have inadvertently done serious damage to their unborn babies.

Pregnant teens who smoke, for example, are injuring their babies. A pregnant teen who drinks is increasing her baby's chances of being born with fetal alcohol syndrome (FAS). Retardation and learning problems are common characteristics of a child born with FAS.

Statistically, teens are more apt to use illegal drugs than adults, and a pregnant teen using such drugs is putting her baby at grave risk. Janie Gore Golan, an investigator of prenatal drug exposure, explains the grim consequences of using crack or cocaine:

> When you use crack or cocaine during a pregnancy, the child you give birth to may at first look fine, healthy and normal. Then a week later, he or she could have the shakes and be irritable. And by irritable, I mean screaming and not able to sleep. Crack babies don't tolerate feedings well. They are extremely demanding. As they grow older and you hug them, they won't hug back. Instead, they go rigid or act like a wet

doll. They are not able to respond or give love in return. There's no comforting these children.[5]

Even if illegal drugs are not part of a pregnant teen's life, pregnant teens are more likely to have engaged in some unhealthy practices. "Even if we're not talking about crack or marijuana," says one counselor, "we're talking about teenagers. They are less worried about things they eat or drink. They might have a cigarette, or a beer, or a wine cooler. Or they pop diet pills. Or they simply don't have the energy or money to make sure they're eating well. You compare the health habits of a fifteen-year-old who doesn't want to be pregnant with those of a 28-year-old who's been trying to have a baby and who's taking the vitamins, getting sleep, eating right—my money's on the 28-year-old."[6]

An uncomfortable subject

Though it is certainly true that teen parents face many difficulties today, teens having babies in the United States is nothing new. American teenagers—married and unmarried—have been having babies for many generations. What has changed, say some, is society's perceptions—not only of teens but of sex.

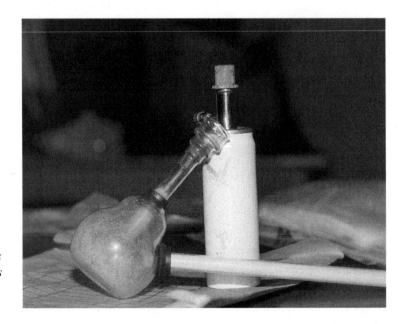

Teenage mothers are more likely than adults are to use illegal drugs like crack during pregnancy.

Up until the 1970s, the subject of sex was taboo, even when talking about a married couple. "You didn't even use the word pregnant," recalls one woman who was a teen in the 1960s. "You said, 'She's in the family way.'"[7]

Society was so uncomfortable with the idea of sex and pregnancy, in fact, that as late as the mid-1970s, married pregnant women were discouraged from teaching in public schools. This was done, explains one sociologist, "lest their swelling bellies cross that invisible boundary separating the real world (where sex and pregnancy existed) from the schools (where they did not)."[8] If society was having trouble feeling comfortable with married pregnant women, it should be no surprise that unmarried pregnant women were viewed with dismay.

"A secret thing"

Through the first half of the twentieth century, a pregnant unmarried teenager and her family were objects of shame, and the young girl was often hurried into a home for unwed mothers or sent on an extended "visit" with a faraway relative until she gave birth. The baby was almost always put up for adoption.

In the poor neighborhoods, unmarried pregnant teens fared no better than their counterparts in upper-class white communities. Louise Eaton was a sixteen-year-old in 1922 and remembers well what it was like to be poor and black in New York: "In my times, if a girl got pregnant and she didn't have a husband, she found one! Or if she remained single, she went into a home. Her pregnancy was a secret thing."[9]

The same attitude prevailed in the 1950s and early 1960s. A teen who married the father of her baby presented no problem for society at all; it was assumed that most women would stay home and be homemakers rather than pursue an outside career. With a husband to support her and her baby, she was neither an object of shame nor an economic burden for society.

"I knew quite a lot of girls who got married young and had children," one woman recalls. "It wasn't a bad thing, nothing unusual. Just hard. And if you were a poor person, there wasn't the kind of help you had today. No welfare, of course. We had to do things on our own."[10]

Things changed

But society began to change in the late 1960s and 1970s, becoming more open about sex and pregnancy. Not only were men and women living together without being married, but many unmarried women were having babies and raising them by themselves. So much had changed, in fact, that among single-parent families in 1992, the largest group consisted of families headed by never-married mothers. In 1970, such families made up only 1 percent of single-parent families.

However, rising prices for life's necessities and salaries that have failed to keep pace have made it impossible for many single parents to support their families without assistance. State and national welfare budgets, already stretched by the numbers of unemployed and working poor, are completely overwhelmed by the number of young mothers who have no means of supporting the babies they are having.

Those who work with teen parents sometimes feel overwhelmed, too. "It just got out of control," says one youth worker at a teen center.

> Too many kids getting pregnant, too few marketable skills. They quit school and then—what? A job flipping hamburgers at McDonald's? For a few hours a day, maybe? And that's providing the baby isn't sick, or the bus is on time, or five or six other things.
>
> And the worst thing about it is that the teens who are having babies now, the ones I'm seeing at the center here, are themselves the children of other teen mothers fourteen or fifteen. Some have boyfriends, very few are married or have prospects for jobs. I'd say we've got us a problem.[11]

1

The Increase in Teen Pregnancy

CERTAINLY THE HIGH rate of pregnant teens in the United States is due to a high rate of sexual activity among teens. Research shows that more than 75 percent of American girls between the ages of fifteen and nineteen are sexually active; in 1970 the number was only 29 percent. There is no one reason for the dramatic increase, say sociologists; rather, it is a combination of factors.

Dysfunctional families

Many teenage mothers—between 80 and 90 percent—come from families in which constant fighting, chemical abuse, alcoholism, or mental illness are common. To escape an unstable home life, some teenage girls are often in a hurry to find intimacy with a caring boy.

"I really mostly wanted to be close," says one fourteen-year-old who has been sexually active for over a year. "I hated being at my house. My mom and dad were always in the middle of some big thing—he'd yell, she'd cry. It was too much. And with Brian, there wasn't any of that—it was just peaceful. I didn't necessarily plan on sleeping with him, but it was okay. And it was a way to get close to someone who cared."[12]

Research also suggests a link between teen pregnancy and a history of sexual abuse. Studies have shown that the majority of sexually active teens have been victims of sexual abuse. As many as 75 percent of teens who become pregnant report that they had been sexually abused earlier in their lives by fathers, stepfathers, or other family members.

Kay, nineteen, was raped repeatedly by her grandfather when she was small, and as a teen who became pregnant at age fifteen, she feels that the abuse played a large role in her own sexual activity. "I did become sexually active early," she admits. "I mean, the father of my child wasn't the first boy I had a relationship with. But I look back on it now, and I think that being raped like that had a lot to do with me starting sex earlier than lots of girls. . . . It's like I skipped other stuff that kids did and went right to that grown-up part, I think."[13]

Where are the parents?

But family dysfunction is not the only contributing factor to teen sexual activity. For many teens, parents are simply not paying attention. "They give their kids way too much freedom, way too much leeway," says one social worker. "They are busy with work or other aspects of their

Many parents become less involved in their child's life during the teenage years.

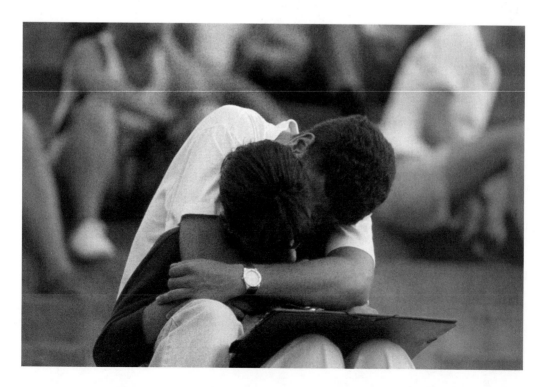

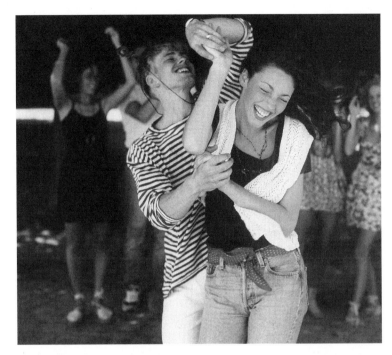

Interaction with friends is a big part of childhood and teenage years. Many teens today learn about sex from friends and classmates rather than from parents.

lives, and they congratulate themselves on being the kind of parents who trust their kids. But in a lot of cases, that's just a way of justifying their own noninvolvement."[14]

Teachers and school counselors notice such noninvolvement long before it gets to the point of teen sex. According to Robyn Cousin, the family coordinator for the Minneapolis public schools, there is a sharp decrease in the amount of parental interest between grade school and junior high. Not only do fewer parents attend school functions and academic conferences, she says, but the parents also cut themselves off from what could be helpful interaction with other parents. Says Cousin, "When we talk with families of adolescents, I'm amazed at the loss of community, networking, and support among parents."[15]

The lack of supervision

The lack of parental supervision is a key factor in the rising number of young teen pregnancies. Whereas in generations gone by, fourteen- and fifteen-year-olds would come home after school to find their mother starting dinner or cleaning house, today far more teens live in single-parent homes in which the mother works fulltime. Even in intact, two-parent families, both parents hold jobs outside the home.

And if parents think that kids are just doing homework or talking on the phone after school, say experts, they are simply kidding themselves. One boy who became a father at sixteen knows that if he and his girlfriend hadn't had the promise of an empty house every afternoon, it most likely wouldn't have happened. "My parents are divorced," he says simply.

> My mom's never here. So when my girlfriend wants to come over, it's cool. No one will bother us. I've heard my dad talk about when he was a teenager and kids went to make-out spots in their cars to have sex. But our way seemed way better—at least it seemed that way until Gloria got pregnant.[16]

"That is sex"

With so many parents spending so little time with their teens, it follows that few are taking the time to talk frankly about the subject of sex. Many parents assume their children are hearing about it at school or from older siblings, and they are reluctant to set—or even talk about—limits or expectations.

What might surprise parents is that, although teens do get a great deal of information from friends or classmates, many would prefer hearing it from their parents. Says one girl, "I got all the information about menstruation and stuff from my friend and her mother. It made me kind of sad, because I wanted to have that talk with my own mom, you know? I think she was just too uncomfortable or something, but I look at it as one more time we didn't connect."[17]

Missed opportunities for parent-child conversations about sex are common, for a variety of reasons. Claims one researcher, "[Parents] either avoid the subject, miss the mark by starting the discussion too long before or after the sexual encounter, or just plain stonewall them."[18]

One seventeen-year-old boy recalls approaching his mother with questions and getting nowhere, probably because she was uncomfortable with the topic. "I was nine when I asked my mother the Big Question," he says. "I'll never forget. She took out her driver's license and pointed to the line about male or female. 'That is sex,' she said."[19]

Another girl recalled a similar experience. "I love my mother, but she never really talked to me, and I don't feel like I can talk to her about private matters. She acts like we shouldn't talk about sex. She only told me after my period, that I shouldn't go with boys."[20]

"It's all mad-sex stuff"

The gaps in the information that teens receive about sex from their parents and their peers are more than filled by the media. From talk shows such as *Jerry Springer* to melodramas like *Dawson's Creek,* from MTV to thousands of CDs, American teens are getting more than a little exposure to frank sexual content. "You can learn a lot from cable," explains one sixteen-year-old. "It's all mad-sex stuff."[21]

A teenage girl watches television in her home. Much of what teens know about sex they learn from television.

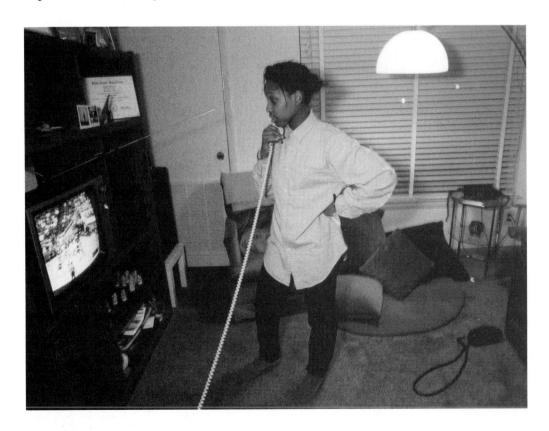

A fourteen-year-old from Denver says that it doesn't matter to him that his parents haven't talked with him about sex, because for years he has been educated by television. "If you watch TV," he explains, "they've got everything you want to know. That's how I learned to kiss, when I was eight. And the girl told me, 'Oh, you sure know how to do it.'"[22]

None of this surprises Jeff Rodriguez, the director of education at Texas's Adolescent Pregnancy Prevention, who notes that television and other media fail to tell the whole story. "No other generation has been exposed to so many media messages about sex," he maintains. "Pick up any CD jacket; you're going to see some really irresponsible messages about having sex. See a movie; the couples are never married, they never talk about contraception or disease or other negative consequences."[23]

The pressure is everywhere

But even in the best circumstances, when teens are informed and have talked with parents about limits, sex is a difficult force to resist—especially when the pressure from peers to have sex is so great. Often, a girl feels as though if she doesn't give in, her boyfriend will no longer be interested in her.

It is estimated that half of all teens who get pregnant were coerced, or pressured, into having sex when they weren't ready. Physician's Associate Virginia Reath says that she sees many teens in her practice and often has what has come to be a very standard conversation:

"Did you initiate the sex?"

The answer: "Not really."

"Did you try to stop it?"

"Yes, but not enough."

"Was it rape?"

"Well, no. It's just easier to do it than to say 'no' and have to fight."[24]

Social workers say such pressure is so severe, and so common, that in a survey of one thousand teenage girls in Atlanta, 84 percent said that what they most wanted to get out of their sex education course was how to say "no." Without an effective way to refuse sexual advances, they say, they felt as though they were alienating any boy they dated.

"I just [had sex] to get it over with," says one fifteen-year-old girl. "My boyfriend had been pressuring me and pressuring me—he told me he only wanted to show me how much he loved me. If I didn't want to have sex with him, he said, how can he know I care about him? Now I know that's a lot of shit, but then it just seemed easier to do it than turn every evening into a fight."[25]

"Because everyone was talking about it"

Interestingly, many teens feel as much, if not more, pressure from their peer group as from their boyfriend or girlfriend. Even though they may have chosen not to engage in sexual activity, strong peer pressure often pushes them into situations where they will compromise their beliefs.

On ABC's television show *Nightline,* a young teen said that young people his age aren't getting the support they need to survive such sexual pressure. "I am a freshman at a very high-class school in California and the pressure I feel to have sex is incredible," he says. "I am not yet ready to have sex, but I almost feel that I need to do so, so this intense amount of pressure is lifted."[26]

Many teens feel pressure from their peers and close friends to become sexually active.

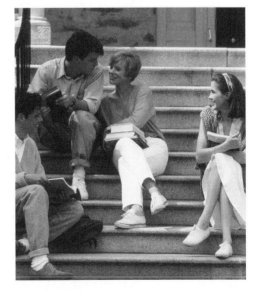

Eighteen-year-old Jeannie, a senior in high school, had decided to wait until marriage to have sex, but as more and more of her friends began to be sexually active, she says, she felt more alone—and less sure of her decision. "Because everyone was talking about it, a part of me started to question my beliefs," she admits. "I started to feel like, 'How come everyone else thinks there's nothing wrong with this? Maybe it's just part of being a teen, and I'm missing out.'"[27]

For boys, the pressure is intense, too; having sex early has become an indication of their maturity or a sign of their masculinity. One high school boy says that, especially on athletic teams, sexual conquests are an indicator of a boy's status:

> If they haven't [had intercourse] then they are like outcasts. Like, "Man, you never made love to a girl!" Some of them get teased a lot. It's like on the baseball team and they start talking about that and you have got the younger guys out there and you could tell because they are all quiet and stuff and they won't talk. Some of the other people start laughing at them and start getting on them and get them kind of upset.[28]

Teens who have given in to the pressure and engaged in sex before they were really ready say that they are sorry they did, for it detracted from the experience. "All of my friends were having sex and I was curious to see what it was all about," one Colorado teen explains. "I didn't even know the guy very well, and I don't even want to know him. It wasn't like it is shown on TV or in the movies. I didn't even enjoy it."[29]

"They keep these stupid ideas alive"

Another reason for the high rate of pregnancy among teens is the lack of sound information teens have about how *not* to get pregnant. Many social workers and counselors are baffled by the kind of misinformation sexually active teens are working with. "Lots of kids act smart, talk like they know about sex," says one social worker.

> But when it comes down to knowing how babies are conceived—they're babies themselves. Even many of the kids who are very sexually active haven't got a clue. They keep these stupid ideas alive, like you can't get pregnant if you have intercourse standing up, or you can't get pregnant the first time you have sex. There are dozens of these ideas, and tens of thousands of babies that are living proof that these ideas are just plain garbage.[30]

Many teens are living in a fantasy world in that they don't believe anything bad will ever happen to them. They feel invulnerable and invincible. As far as sex goes, they imagine that the chances of becoming pregnant are so infinitesimal that they simply don't worry about it. Counselors say that this "charmed life" idea is one of the

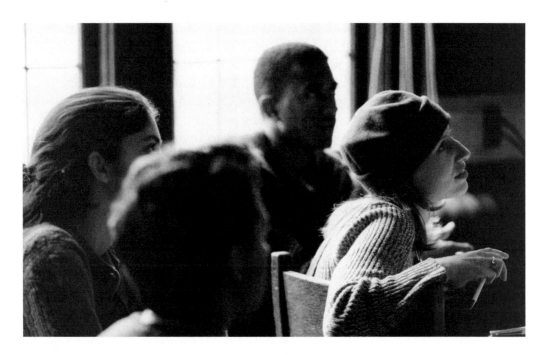

reasons that only two or three out of every ten sexually active teens use birth control.

Nineteen-year-old Mary admits that she belongs to this category of teen mothers. "I never worried about getting pregnant," she says. "I wasn't on birth control, and he never used a condom. I guess we just figured we'd be lucky, so we didn't think about it too much. Besides," she says as an afterthought, "my friend Colleen had sex a lot more often than I did, and she'd never gotten pregnant."[31]

Some teens believe that somehow pregnancy is something that only happens to others. One girl recalls feeling that she simply wasn't "the type" of girl who got pregnant, so she didn't worry about it. "You hear about it happening," she says, "but the girls who get pregnant are *stupid*. They're sluts. They're the ones always in trouble. I wasn't doing drugs. I wasn't out drinking. So why would I worry about getting pregnant? That's how I thought."[32]

"I remembered that I'd missed a few days"

However, it is not enough simply to be aware that sex carries a real risk of pregnancy and to know that birth control is

Although health education is often taught in school, many teens who engage in sexual intercourse remain misinformed about how not to become pregnant.

important. Many teens who use birth control find that it has failed them—and they, too, become pregnant.

One problem is that, regardless of the method of birth control, there are no 100 percent guarantees, even when birth control devices are used correctly. And often the birth control methods are not correctly used. Condoms, one of the most frequently used forms of birth control used by teens, are effective only *most* of the time. Researchers say that between 10 and 18 percent of teens relying on condoms become pregnant.

Sometimes a teen reuses a condom or uses it with a petroleum-based lubricant that can dissolve the condom's latex. This lack of knowledge about how to use a condom effectively, experts say, and the lack of motivation to use one every time mean that condoms fail to prevent pregnancy much more often.

Birth control pills, too, are only effective if taken correctly—which means taken consistently each cycle. Kay, who became pregnant during her freshman year of high school, felt confident having a sexual relationship with her boyfriend because she was on the pill. When a routine school exam showed that she was pregnant, she had to rethink her use of the pills. "When I thought back," she admits, "I remembered that I'd missed a few days. That was what did it, I guess."[33]

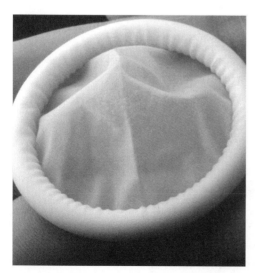

Common birth control products like this condom are effective only if properly used. Many teen pregnancies occur because of improper use of birth control devices.

Embarrassment and other excuses

Some teens would say that the main problem with birth control was procuring it in the first place. Many people, horrified by the rate of teen pregnancy, ask why young people aren't using birth control. What they don't always remember is that, for many teenagers, getting birth control is a daunting experience.

For girls, it means they must get in the medical system—have a complete gynecological exam, which most have never had—and talk to a doctor face-to-face about wanting birth control. Though no medical OK is necessary for boys, sometimes even buying a package of condoms can be difficult. "Even if it's only a male going to the store to get condoms," says one clinic worker, "he has to put up with comments like, 'I'll have to charge you an entertainment tax.' A female goes in and she hears, 'Hey, honey, you're not the one who's supposed to be buying these.' She gets embarrassed."[34]

Brad, a young sexually active teen, knew he should be using birth control. However, because he lived in a small town, he was embarrassed to buy condoms at a store close by. He was temporarily saved when a friend offered to get him some at a doctor's clinic.

> He grabbed a whole handful for me. And that was great, for awhile. But then, when the supply ran out, I stopped using them. See, it was real uncomfortable for me to just go out and buy them myself, like in a drugstore, or whatever. If I went to the Festival or another store around here, everyone would know what I was doing. It's a pretty small town, and that would be embarrassing. I kind of felt real dumb doing that.[35]

Pregnant on purpose

A final reason why some teens get pregnant may surprise a lot of people: In some instances teens *want* to have a child. Research done by the Alan Guttmacher Institute in New York indicates that approximately 15 percent of teen pregnancies are intentional. With so much attention being paid to the problems faced by teen parents, why would an unmarried teen choose to have a child?

One reason is that many teenage girls who become pregnant feel that something is missing in their lives. Perhaps they don't get along well with their parents, don't do well in school, or don't have dreams for the future. A baby provides them with a way out of the house, a way to begin their own lives.

The idea of a baby, of some little person to love and who would love them, seems intriguing too. Explains one youth worker, "These girls are motivated by the idea that having a baby will give them the love or sense of hope they feel is missing."[36]

"I was feeling so insecure about everything," one pregnant sixteen-year-old admits. "I thought being pregnant and having a cute little baby to hold would make me feel better."[37]

Youth workers stress that such fantasies are just that—fantasies. "Girls who think this way are forgetting that these are not dolls that they can put down when they're tired of dressing them and changing their diapers," says one social worker. "They get intrigued by the commercials

The care of babies requires enormous energy and time. Many teenage mothers are both unprepared for and incapable of providing the attention babies need.

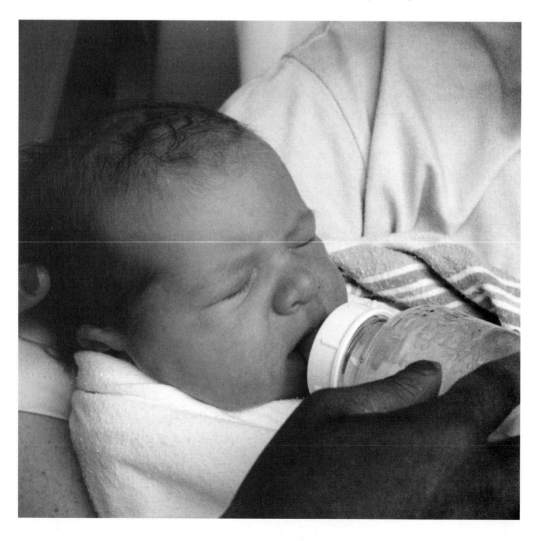

for baby food or diapers. They ooh and ahh, but I tell them, 'That's not what having a baby is.' But I know they don't really believe me."[38]

Peer approval

Some youth workers report that, among girls, pregnancy is often viewed as a sign of maturity or femininity. One doctor in the middle-class community of Tipton, Indiana, says, "Teen pregnancy is not looked poorly upon by peers here. In fact, it's greeted with a great deal of excitement." The taboos associated with being single and pregnant, some say, have become totally reversed among teens, and that attitude has this doctor worried. Although in many ways it is good that schools are helping pregnant teens by offering on-campus day care and parenting classes, he says, he worries that such things may encourage teens to choose pregnancy, thereby increasing its status among the high school students. "There is this mixed message that the community is sending,"[39] he says.

Wanting to stay together

Some teens hope that being pregnant will give them a sort of hold on their boyfriends, who they fear might be losing interest in them. A girl might think that when she is pregnant, the boy will stay with her—maybe even marry her—and protect her and her baby.

Those who counsel teens advise against this sort of reasoning. A teen who gets pregnant by neglecting to take her birth control pills, for example, is being untruthful to her boyfriend, say counselors, and it demeans the baby down to the role of a sort of insurance policy. "It's a bad way to operate," says one counselor. "It's bad to start any relationship off with lies or deceit, and here some kids start a whole life off that way."[40]

Unfortunately for many teen girls who intentionally get pregnant for this reason, the boy rarely lives up to their idealized expectations. Some leave immediately after hearing the news; others might stay until the baby is born. Not many remain too long afterwards, as one teen found out.

I expected commitment of just being a father. Of being there saying, "I'm going to help you. I'll be there to take care of Jimmy when you want, when you need to do other things." I expected his support emotionally, financially, as much as he could. I expected him to be there for me. . . . I expected him to love me because I was the woman who had his baby. But he loves everyone else who didn't.[41]

2

"What Do I Do Now?"

IN MANY CASES, even when a teen is aware of the risks when she becomes sexually active, pregnancy is a surprise. How a girl learns she is pregnant—and the kinds of stress she endures in breaking the news to her family, as well as to the father of the baby—is often traumatic.

Finding out by accident

For many teens who have tried to minimize the risk of pregnancy, the early physical indications that they are pregnant are so unexpected, so subtle, that they are completely ignored. Being overly tired or feeling bloated or nauseated can be chalked up to a number of ailments—from the flu to premenstrual cramping.

Health care professionals are often bewildered when girls come in several months pregnant without any knowledge of what is happening to them. In many cases, they request treatment for something quite different, but a routine question on the medical form prompts some follow-up.

Mary learned she was pregnant by accident. She had gone to the emergency room for a strep test; having had a very sore throat for more than a week, she decided to see a doctor. A nurse was helping her fill out the paperwork. It was easy, until a particular question came up. "Well, the one question about when my last period was had me stumped," she recalls. "I thought for a while and decided it was August. And this was October, when I was filling this out. The nurse saw that, and asked me if I wanted a pregnancy test, and I figured I should."[42]

Another girl was having an X ray to see if she had pneumonia and noticed a sign in the technician's office that said, "If you are pregnant or think you might be pregnant, tell us." Although she was almost sure she was not pregnant, she was sexually active, so she asked the doctor to do a pregnancy test—without letting her mother know. "I can still see it to this day," she says. "As I walked out of the doctor's office, he flashed a piece of paper. On it was the word 'positive.' I got in the car and cried."[43]

"Sort of positive"

Many pregnant teens, however, suspect that they are pregnant before a doctor makes the diagnosis. A missed or unusually light period is almost always the first clue, and means that a pregnancy test is a good idea.

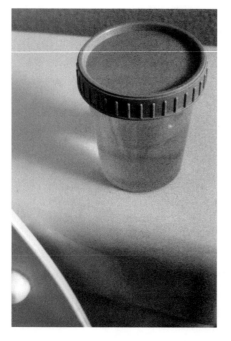

Home pregnancy tests like this one can be expensive, inaccurate, and difficult to read.

Often teens will purchase a home pregnancy test so that they can avoid an expensive or potentially embarrassing trip to a doctor's office or clinic. The problem, though, is that the results are not always easy to interpret. Jessica, sixteen, was concerned because she'd skipped a period. The following month she had what she calls "an odd period"—very light and unusually free of cramping. Her boyfriend, Jason, remembers that the home pregnancy tests were both expensive and ambivalent—and Jessica had used two of them. "She'd taken one the month before . . . but that test was negative. But [the second one] came out sort of positive. I say 'sort of' because the strip was supposed to turn pink, but it didn't come out the same color as on the box. It was a real light, light pink. So we still didn't know."[44]

Secrecy

Even in cases in which the home test is clearly positive, a teen's next step should be to verify the results with a doctor. Teens are usually very apprehensive about such an office visit, so they tend to avoid their regular clinic or family doctor. "No way I wanted to see my doctor," remembers one teen. "He was the one who delivered me, delivered my brothers. I know there's supposed to be some doctor-patient confidence thing, where they can't tell. But what if he forgot and mentioned to my mom sometime, 'Yeah, I saw Katy today—she's upset about being pregnant.' No way I want to do that!"[45]

In some cases, however, because of insurance company rules, clinics require parental permission to do tests or blood work on minors. Then a teen is often faced with the additional humiliation of having to lie. Lisa, a Native American teen, went to her doctor's office but was told they couldn't see her because her mother wasn't with her.

> I didn't have a slip or anything that was signed by a parent, so I had to tell them a big old lie. When they told me I had to go home to have a permission slip signed, I told them my mother was working and [I] couldn't reach her. I told them she was cleaning a house, and I had no idea what the phone number was. Really, I just didn't want to have her come with me.[46]

Finding out

Because so many teen pregnancies are unplanned, it is not surprising that the reaction of the mother-to-be is usually one of shock or disbelief. Some teens cry or leave the clinic in a daze after a brief visit with the doctor. Doctors say that the worry they hear from teens most often is "How will I tell my boyfriend?" or, even worse, "What will my parents say?"

Few things are as painful to share with parents as the news of an unplanned pregnancy. The news is sometimes seen by parents as a betrayal—an admission of sexual activity when perhaps the teen had insisted there was none, for example. An announcement of pregnancy is also a signal that life will take a very different path from the one both teens and parents had envisioned. School, career, participation in high school activities—all of these will either disappear for the time being or change dramatically.

Many teens who have gone through the ordeal say that there is no way of accurately predicting how parents will react to the news. Some parents who are ordinarily very supportive often are so disappointed and surprised at first that they are unable to offer any support to their pregnant daughters.

After she had just turned fifteen, Kay had to tell her parents she was pregnant. The shock and anger from her mother were predictable, she says, but her father was the real surprise. "I was dreading telling him," she says. "We had always been so close. He didn't know I was sexually active, either. I felt like I was letting him down. I was afraid to face him, but I really thought he'd be supportive of me. I was wrong. I told him in the car, when we were coming home from dinner one night. He was so mad—it was like I was really on my own. He said, 'Boy, Kay, you did this and you're going to suffer for it.' That was really hard on me."[47]

"I didn't have anybody to count on"

The parents of eighth-grader Safa had a similar reaction to her news. Her mother, she says, wouldn't even discuss it, because "she'd always expected it of me." And her father, a devout Muslim, was furious. After telling her that she had betrayed her name, which is an Islamic word for "purity," he called her a tramp and refused to help her any further. Safa says she had never felt so desperate, so alone. "I didn't have anybody to count on," she says. "And I was having this baby."[48]

Counselors say that the anticipation of such reactions by parents often makes teens unwilling to talk to their families. Feeling as though they have let down or humiliated their parents adds to their own feelings of sadness and confusion. In some cases pregnant girls experience depression and even consider suicide.

Suicidal feelings

"I wasn't the first in our family to get herself pregnant," says eighteen-year-old Jodi.

When I was fourteen, I got pregnant by a friend of a friend, at a party. As soon as I found out I was pregnant, I knew I should tell my mom. In fact, I *wanted* to tell her, to have her tell me things would work out. But I didn't, because I'd been there when my parents heard this same news from my older sister just six months before. And my mom and dad were so sad—I'd never seen my dad cry before. I couldn't do that to them! I started thinking I should just kill myself, and I thought a lot about it, nearly every day. It was the lowest I'd ever felt in my whole life.[49]

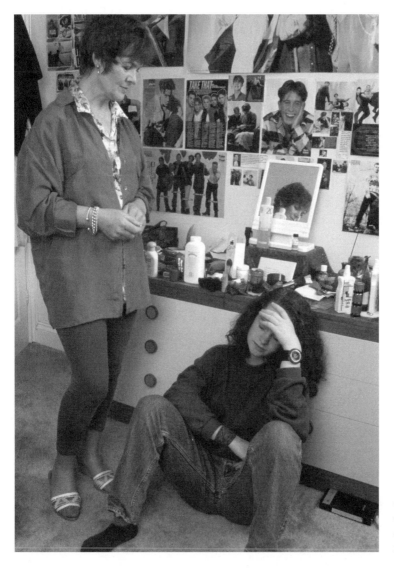

Parents often react with disappointment and anger to the news that their child is pregnant.

Social workers stress to teens that there are always options and that their parents' first reactions—no matter how painful—will usually mellow in time. Even if parents insist on being unhelpful or angry, other family members or counselors can often help by offering support.

Boyfriends

There are differing reactions from boyfriends, just as there are from parents. Some boys are thrilled that they have fathered a child, believing that impregnating a young woman somehow makes them men. Especially among boys from low-income families, who may have limited goals for the future, the idea of helping create a child is a source of pride. Such an attitude may help a pregnant teen feel that at least someone is on her side.

However, many boys are disinterested or, even worse, hostile. When confronted with a pregnancy, the young man may demand proof that the child belongs to him or ask how his girlfriend knows that it is his child. Social workers say such reactions are very common and are often the result of fear, rather than any real belief that they aren't the father.

"Lots of young men have a very limited idea of what it takes to be a father. After the sex, they sort of tune out," says one counselor. "And here comes a girlfriend, telling him he's going to be a father. What's expected of him? Marriage? Money? Responsibility? Those are scary alternatives to the life he is living, and not nearly as much fun."[50]

A quiet abortion

Expecting anger from her parents and sensing disinterest from her boyfriend, a pregnant teen is often in the position of making very difficult choices on her own. For teens who are anxious to hide their pregnancy from family and friends, an abortion may at first seem to be the best choice. In fact, in 1996 researchers estimated that 401,500 teens opted to end their pregnancies this way—only slightly fewer than the number of teens who decided to keep their babies.

"We counsel teens when they reach the stage of having to choose," says one social worker. "It's important that girls understand all of the facts before they go through something like abortion. Many see it as sort of a cure-all— a simple procedure that when done, restores their lives to their pre-pregnant state. And that is not always the case."[51]

Abortion, while a relatively safe procedure when done in a clinic or hospital, can still be traumatic for some who undergo it. Many young women find that having an abortion made them feel guilty and sad, and for some, even years later, the feelings haven't gone away.

A nurse prepares a patient for an abortion. Some pregnant teens choose to have abortions rather than give birth.

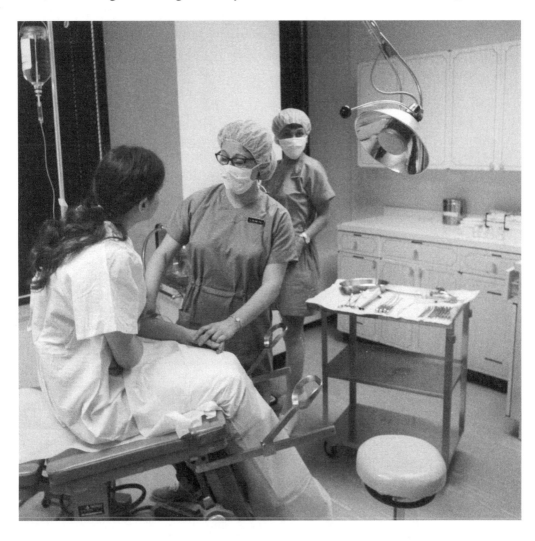

"It was probably best for me at the time," says one college sophomore. "But I don't look back on that time with anything but regret. I feel bad, and I'm not sure why. I was able to keep going to high school, and my life was not disrupted with a baby when I was fifteen. But I feel kind of melancholy, like it was a no-win thing."[52]

"I saw a swing set"

Some teens reject abortion for those same reasons. Whether for religious or emotional reasons, they feel that abortion is the wrong choice for them. Interestingly, many teens have every intention of having an abortion, but back out at the last minute because the idea makes them uncomfortable.

Donna, seventeen, says she had her boyfriend drive her to a clinic one Saturday morning. She had enough money for the procedure, and although she wasn't looking forward to it, she had convinced herself it was the right thing to do. But just before they arrived at the clinic, she says, she had second thoughts.

"I looked out the car window, and I saw a swing set," she says, shrugging. "I know that sounds weird, but it made me think. I wondered about this baby, and it made me sad that he or she would never grow up to swing, or have a sandbox, or anything."

"And it was my decision—I was the one that was depriving the baby of a life. I ended up telling Brad to turn the car around, and I told my parents about being pregnant. I ended up giving my daughter up for adoption—hopefully to some nice family that will buy her a swing set!"[53]

Too late, too difficult

Some teens find that, although they have no problem with the idea of having an abortion, they lack the money to afford one. Occasionally, a boyfriend may offer to help out, but unless parents are told and are willing to help, such a procedure can be beyond the resources of some teens.

Other times, teens do not find out that they are pregnant until they are too far along to safely have an abortion. After

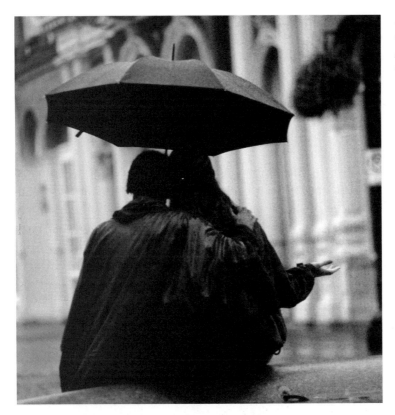

Determining what to do about an unplanned pregnancy can be an agonizing decision.

telling her boyfriend and getting no support from him, Kay decided to abort her pregnancy. She was unwilling to tell her parents, so she and two friends planned a trip to a clinic north of the city where she lived. The friends got up at five on Saturday morning and endured a long bus ride.

"None of us really knew how to get there," she recalls, "so it was kind of stressful. They were trying to be really loyal, but all I felt was nervousness. I didn't want to think too much about what I was doing, you know?"

"Anyway, when we got to the clinic, I found out I was late. I mean, not late for my appointment, but late in my pregnancy. I was three months along, and that changed everything. The clinic could still do the abortion, but it would be more complicated, and way more expensive."

Kay decided not to make another appointment at the clinic. "I guess I had an option," she says sadly. "I could have made another appointment and come back again. But all I wanted . . . was to just go home and go to bed. I was crying and stressed out and nervous. I just wanted to go home to my own room and cry."[54]

Too much trouble

A final reason why some teens reconsider having an abortion is the red tape involved. Although laws differ from state to state, the majority of states require that parents must sign a consent form before a minor child can have an abortion. If a teen does not want to inform her parents, she can appear before a judge who, after hearing her situation, can sign a release saying that the abortion can legally take place.

A pregnant teenager who comes from a state where such laws apply will often decide against having an abortion. After all, one of the reasons cited most often for having an abortion is that it can allow a girl to end a pregnancy while keeping it secret from her family and friends.

"I thought abortion was legal, but it isn't really," says Jennifer, sixteen. "I mean, it isn't available to me where I live, unless I tell both of my parents or go before a judge. Only if I was married or I was eighteen would it be legal for me to decide on an abortion myself. I guess if I was pregnant, I'd just bite the bullet and tell my folks. I mean, you really can't get around it now, right?"[55]

The least-chosen option

One might think that teens who do not choose abortion but who were not planning on being teenage parents would decide on giving up their baby for adoption. However, only about 3 percent of pregnant teens make that choice.

Many teens who end up keeping their babies said that they saw only abortion—never adoption—as the alternative. Experts say there are several reasons why a teen might prefer to keep her baby rather than put it up for adoption. The most important reason is that the social stigma of being a single mother is not as strong as in decades past. "Whereas just thirty years ago the single, never-married mother was something of an oddity," explains one sociologist, "now women of all ages are choosing to live as single mothers."[56]

"Sure, I thought about it"

One of the most important reasons for giving up a baby in years past was to make sure the child got advantages that the teenage mother could never provide. Today, however, many teens feel that the unconditional love—together with a strong sense of family ties—they can provide the child more than compensates for a lack of material advantages.

Many teens also feel that if they go through the stress and trials of pregnancy and childbirth, keeping the baby is their just "reward." "Sure, I thought about [adoption], but I could never do it," says one sixteen-year-old. "I know a lot of people could do a better job than me of being a mother and they can't get pregnant, but that's not my fault. I'm not going to go through nine months and then give someone else the benefit."[57]

A sixteen-year-old mother kisses her son on the playground. Instead of turning to options like adoption, many teens choose to raise their child on their own.

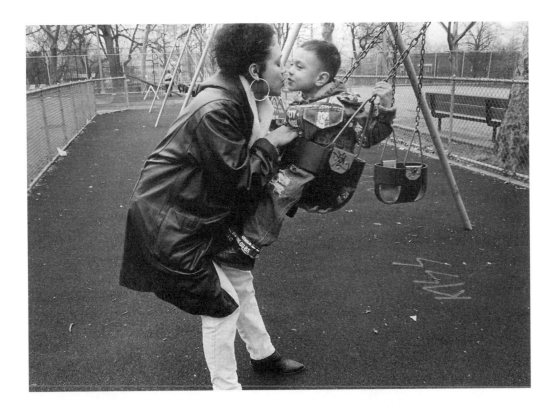

Many teens also worry that having been put up for adoption might make their child feel bad later on. For example, some expectant teens worry that their child will be raised by a couple whose race or ethnicity is different from the child's. Though many states try to match black children with black couples, for example, some black teens worry that their baby will be raised in a white home.

"It's nothing racist, I don't mean that," says one black teen. "But I don't want no baby of mine talking white, acting white. There's a lot that's good about being black, finding out your roots. More schools are doing that now. What roots does a black kid have in a white suburban family? And it won't be that family's fault, because what would they know about it?"[58]

Support to keep their children

Even with a lack of interest from the fathers of their babies, unmarried teens are deciding—in record numbers—to raise their babies themselves. One reason, say experts, is that for teens who are leaning toward keeping their babies, there are a number of support systems in place that can help.

One such support is the welfare system. While there are some who harshly criticize single mothers on welfare—even to the point of accusing them of having babies just to collect a more substantial check each month—few can argue with the fact that a welfare check makes the financial burden of a baby easier for a single teen mother to bear.

Nineteen-year-old Quara applied for welfare right after her child was born. Now she pays about $60 in rent and uses the rest of her check to cover formula, diapers, and other supplies for the baby. Without that check, she admits, she would be lost. "I'm struggling," she says. "The money is not for us, it's [for] our children. It's hard enough trying to depend on the baby's daddy. I really need the AFDC [Aid to Families with Dependent Children]."[59]

Another, more personal, support system is the teen's family. In some cases, a teen's mother might be enthusiastic about a baby in the family, even though at first she might have been angry about her daughter's getting pregnant. As the birth nears, or sometimes after the birth, the teen's mother might actually look forward to helping her daughter raise the child.

Knowing that her own mother can be a source of help is a great relief to a young mother. Not only is there the promise of a safety net when money is tight, but there is a person who can provide information and guidance on taking care of a baby.

"My mother was even kind of excited," admits Yolanda, fifteen. "At first she was mad when I told her I was pregnant, but she got over it fast. She was into getting baby clothes and getting everything ready. I was really glad, too, because I didn't want to do this on my own."[60]

Challenges ahead

A family who is willing to help with a new baby is a real asset, especially when the new mother is a single teenager. While the discomfort and stress a pregnant teen faces is often very difficult, the object of all of this controversy and change—the baby—will add even more stress. When it makes its appearance, the teen is going to need every amount of support and guidance she can get. "The challenges," says one counselor, "just grow and grow."[61]

3

The Challenges of Parenthood

MANY TEENAGERS SAY they feel as though their pregnancy lasts forever, that they feel heavy and tired and that they can't remember what it's like *not* to feel that way. They look forward to the birth of the baby, hoping that they will feel better and have more energy. Having a new baby to introduce to family and friends is something they anticipate, too. Recalls Diana, age seventeen,

> I was eager to get to the hospital. I remembered visiting my Aunt Marcia when she had her baby—I was twelve, I think. And it was fun—she had about ten bouquets of flowers around her room, and my uncle was sitting there, real proud. People would come and bring presents for the baby, and it was so cool.

> I wasn't really looking forward to the pain of childbirth—I knew that was supposed to be bad—but the afterwards part I was really looking forward to. I just kept telling myself, after April 12 [her due date] everything will be fine.[62]

Reality

However, the reality faced by teens after they give birth is often much different from their expectations. Childbirth is usually painful and difficult, and most mothers are physically and emotionally drained by the time the baby is born.

"I was happy, yeah," remembers one girl. "But I was so out of it. I couldn't believe I didn't even have the energy to keep my eyes open. I don't remember much at all, except my mom telling me that the baby was healthy. I didn't even know it was a girl until the next morning when the nurse brought her in. And by then she was like ten hours old!"[63]

Of course, expectations and reality often don't match. Another teen says she was disappointed in the way the baby looked, and that made her sad. "He was so wrinkly and red-looking," she remembers. "I wanted him to be cute and everything. He just slept and looked like a little shriveled-up old man. I kept thinking, 'How come everyone else got cute babies?'"[64]

"I don't even love her"

The unrealistic expectations that teens have, along with the changes in the balance of their hormones, can result in depression. Sometimes this begins a week or two after delivery, while other teens say they feel sad and alone almost right away. Postpartum depression, as this condition is called, can affect a new mother of any age, but it is often fueled by the unhappiness or stress a teen mother may be feeling before the birth.

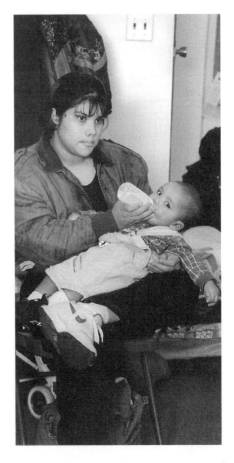

Faced with the stress of becoming a parent, teen mothers often become depressed soon after their child's birth.

"Maybe she's angry that the father didn't come to the hospital to see the baby, or maybe she's afraid of what kind of mother she'll be," says one counselor. "There are so many things that affect a new mom, and teens are often the most vulnerable. And if *they* are feeling vulnerable, they look at the baby, and—goodness! They think, 'I'm supposed to be responsible for this little life?' Without strong family ties or a committed husband or boyfriend, this can be a very lonely time."[65]

Kay, nineteen, says that she wasn't surprised that she felt depressed when her daughter was born, because she had been sad before the birth. Her boyfriend had expressed almost no interest in the idea of a baby, and her parents were less than supportive.

"She was a pretty little baby," says Kay, "but I really didn't have much feeling for her one way or another. I admit it. When she was first born, I said to my mom, 'I don't even love her.' She told me not to worry, that everyone feels that way when they first have a baby. I don't know if she was just saying that to make me feel better, or what. I cried, because it didn't seem right not to love her. . . . I wasn't excited, or happy, or anything. It just seemed like a lot of work."[66]

"I felt kind of guilty"

Safa had the same reaction when her son was born. The baby's father had shown very little interest in forming a lasting relationship with her, and her own parents were equally unsupportive. She knew that her reaction to the baby was temporary, she says, but it bothered her all the same.

> I didn't love him right away. Not at all. I felt kind of guilty, too. I had a feeling something must be wrong for me not to have those feelings that you'd expect to have when you first see your own child. . . . Terry [the baby's father] didn't come to the hospital to see me or the baby, and that hurt. I know the baby picked up on all of that hurt, that worry. In every picture you could just see the stress in that baby's face, he was so unhappy. It was like he knew what he was getting into, being born.[67]

Crying babies

Despite all the difficulties, there are many teens who find that a baby is a source of great joy. They enjoy showing the baby off to visitors and family and look forward to taking the baby home from the hospital to begin their lives together.

However, social service workers say that when the teen and her baby get home, they face some of the greatest challenges. Whereas the hospital staff was helpful and willing to assist the teen mother in caring for the newborn baby, life outside the hospital is far different. There are no nurses or aides to bathe the baby or to whisk it back to the nursery after a feeding. And although a teen who is living at home may find eager family volunteers to hold a happy baby, those same volunteers are not as willing at three in the morning when the baby is fussy and crying.

"You just can't believe how much babies cry," says Samantha, fifteen. "It's funny how on TV when they show babies, they're always laughing and cooing and stuff. They just don't want to stop sometimes, no matter how much you feed them, or how often you change their diaper. It's the part of being a mother I hate the most, listening to her crying."[68]

A new routine

Whether it is dealing with a fussy baby or getting up during the night (sometimes several times) for feedings, teens learn quickly that life as they knew it before has radically changed. Counselors say that learning to put another person first is a great step toward maturity—but a step that is difficult for many teens to learn, in part because they are going through so many changes that are part of adolescence.

"Teenagers are basically self-absorbed," says one therapist. "That's their very nature; it's what comes with the age. They are pulling away from their own parents, trying

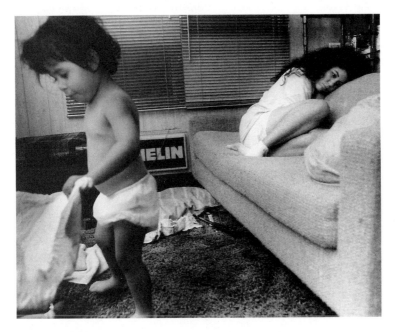

A seventeen-year-old mother watches her two-year-old daughter. Constantly watching out for another person is a task many teens are unprepared for.

to assert their independence in a hundred different ways, and often making a mess of things. That's normal; it's growing up. But you can't be self-absorbed all the time and be a good parent. You've got to be there when the baby needs you, not when you feel like it. And if it means no sleep, then that's that. It's a real growing-up lesson, and a hard one."[69]

Struggles with parents

Another challenge teen parents are often confronted with is the changing relationship with their own parents. Teen parents—especially those who continue to live at home—often complain that their parents continue to treat them as children.

Sarah, sixteen, felt that as long as she was in her mother's house, she would always be treated like a little girl. Even though she has a newborn baby of her own, she says, her mother treats her as though she knows nothing about being a parent.

"If I say the baby's hungry, she'll say, 'It's too soon to feed him,'" complains Sarah. "If I want to go outside and sit on the porch with him, she's like, 'You can't take a baby out in this wind.' It really gets on my nerves."[70]

Too much help

Sometimes teens feel as though their parents are trying to take over the role of being the baby's caregiver. Lisa, sixteen, often asked her mother to babysit her toddler; her mother, she says, was glad to do it. But Lisa noticed that her son behaved badly when she returned to him, and she held her mother responsible.

"When he comes back from [her mother's house], he calls me Lisa, not Mommy," she says angrily. "I hate that. And I know my mom is teaching him that; she gets him to call her Mom and me Lisa. . . . Even when I'm over there, she'll pull that . . .do it right in front of me. She'll say to him, 'Say Lisa,' and she'll point to me. I don't know why she does that."[71]

Another teen mother agrees. She felt her authority had been stripped from her hours after the delivery, when her boyfriend's mother came to the hospital. "When I woke up from the medicine they'd given me [during the delivery], the baby already had a name," she says, her voice breaking. "Tony [the baby's father] had named her Jasmine, and his mother had given her the middle name of Noel, since it was Christmas." In addition, she says, they gave the baby her boyfriend's last name, which made her angry. "That seemed wrong, and it still seems wrong now," she says. "The way things are, with Tony not being a part of her life at all, why should she have his name and not mine? The whole decision was made when I was sleeping, after she was born."[72]

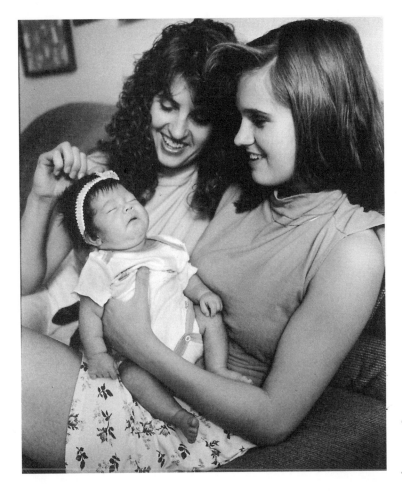

Some teen parents have the good fortune of receiving loving parental support.

Too little help

On the other hand, many teen parents feel that a lack of help makes their lives more stressful. Some wish their parents would offer to do more, such as baby-sit occasionally so that they could go out in the evening with friends.

Others, frustrated at the lack of "time for themselves" that they had before becoming pregnant, wish that their parents could just take control. One girl finds the $300 per month that her father gives her to be inadequate. Although she admits it is selfish, she is irritated that her mother won't raise the baby, as some of her friends' mothers do, so that she could go back to being a "regular teenager."

"Some of these girls . . . I'm serious, they were twelve, thirteen, and fourteen years old, and had two kids! . . . But they got lots of help, usually. Their moms or grandmas raise the kids; the girls just keep doing what they've always done. . . . Hey I wish I could go out drinking every night and sleep in until one o'clock the next afternoon. That's the life I wish I had."[73]

No social life

With or without parental help, however, most teen parents complain that the social life they once had is gone. Often it's simply a matter of time and energy. Friends who want to go out for an evening movie, for example, don't understand that even if a teen parent has access to a baby-sitter, by evening she's usually exhausted from a long day of parenting.

"I'm up early—at least by six," says one mother. "I'm running around all day taking care of Larissa, going to school from noon till four, and by six I'm done. A lot of times I'm too tired to stay awake for the news at ten."[74]

Kay agrees; she says that ever since her daughter was born, she spends almost all of her time with her. "What I *would* like to do is go to a party or hang out with my friends—do stuff with people my own age. . . . But usually I'm home with Jasmine."[75]

Nothing in common

There is another reason why teen parents often feel so isolated from their former friends: They have little in common. Before the teen became pregnant, her life was probably very similar to that of her friends. She went to school and had a boyfriend. Maybe she played on a school sports team or had a part-time job. But the minute she found out she was pregnant, her life changed. If her boyfriend decided to be supportive and involved, his life changed, too. The kinds of things that before might have seemed interesting and exciting to soon-to-be teen parents now often seem like a part of childhood.

When Jason and Jessica had their baby boy, they noticed a big change in their relationship with friends. Jason admits that he has been disappointed by his friends' lack of interest in what has become the most important part of his life—his infant son.

Many teen parents find that they no longer have very much in common with their peers.

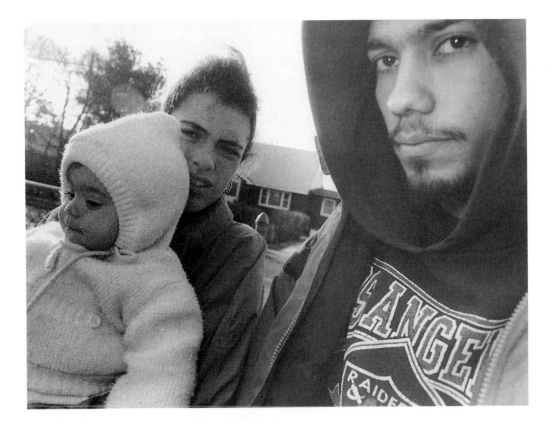

We don't have much of anything to talk about now. They're mostly my age, but it's like we're from two different generations. Like, they're not interested that much in Tyler. They don't come out and say anything, but it's just that they look bored when I'll tell them about funny things Tyler does or if he's getting a new tooth or something.

I know that they think it's really strange that I'm a father now. I don't think they really know how to deal with it. . . . [Jessica and I] make a conscious effort not to talk that much about Tyler when we're out with those friends.[76]

Money is tight

One of the most difficult things about being a teen parent is the financial burden it places on the teen. If a teen mother lives with her parents and they are willing to shoulder the costs of her and the baby, that's great, say teens. But otherwise, it is a constant battle to make ends meet.

"It's one thing to be hungry yourself," says Debbie, eighteen. "I can go without a real meal—just snacking, you know? But you can't tell a baby, 'Hey, go easy on the Pampers, we're broke.' Or 'Don't drink so much formula.' I mean, I figure that baby didn't ask to be born, it was my decision to have her. So I've got to do right by her, make sure she has enough."[77]

But that is difficult for a single mother. Everything for babies costs money—baby clothes, diapers, formula, a stroller—not to mention rent, food, transportation costs, and other necessities. These things would strain almost any family's budget, so it's no wonder that finances are almost always rated as the number-one worry of teen parents.

"I don't know what I'll do"

"I go to sleep at night worrying about how I'm going to get through the next month," says one sixteen-year-old. "And that's how I wake up the next morning, worrying. I don't know if I'll be able to pay off my credit cards, which I've been using for food down at the grocery store. Prices keep going up, but I don't have any more money to spend."[78]

Even with help from welfare or other agencies, young parents struggle. One obvious solution to financial problems is getting a job, but many teens find that that too is difficult. Because they lack a high school diploma and the skills to get a better job, they are almost always stuck in minimum-wage positions with no fringe benefits such as health insurance. In addition, they must weigh in the costs of child care—a consideration that many say makes working too expensive.

"I'd be losing money on the deal," says one girl with a shrug. "I'd be paying a lady more money to watch my baby than I'd be bringing home, once you figure in the bus ride every day. I don't know what I'll do."[79]

A tough job

Not only is it expensive to raise a child, but it is often trying. Babies and young children need constant attention and close supervision. A teen who has not often been around toddlers might be astonished to realize how big a job such supervision is.

Children naturally test boundaries and are bound to get into mischief. Jamie complains that her three-year-old scribbled crayon marks on a freshly painted bedroom wall. Angie is mad because her son has temper tantrums whenever they are in a grocery store. And Safa is furious because her two-year-old has ruined her VCR by sticking a piece of American cheese inside it. Says one young mother,

> You know, I don't know how anyone has the patience to do this all day. How could someone teach preschool is what I want to know. I mean, ten or fifteen of them at once? No way.
>
> I can't imagine having anything nice again—everything I own either has spit-up milk on it or baby food stains. Or she's taken a marker to it, like my purse here—see that? I don't want to spend no money because it will look like trash tomorrow.[80]

A serious challenge

Irritation and frustration are part of every parent's life; very few things can go as smoothly as planned. Experts say that one of the most serious challenges facing teen parents is the potential for abusing their children. In fact, according to a study by sociologists Robert M. Goerge and Bong Joo Lee, a sixteen- or seventeen-year-old mother is nearly 50 percent more likely than a twenty-one-year-old to abuse her child to the point that the child will need to be placed in foster care. For a younger mother of fourteen or fifteen, the likelihood is more than twice that of a twenty-one-year-old mother.

Such figures do not surprise social workers, who say that while some teens make fine parents, it is true that many lack the maturity to care for a child. "They're children themselves," says one counselor. "They don't have the tools yet to make good decisions. They don't deal with frustration well yet. And that's often what it boils down to—how they cope."[81]

Teens often lack the maturity and patience required to deal with small children and sometimes resort to violence.

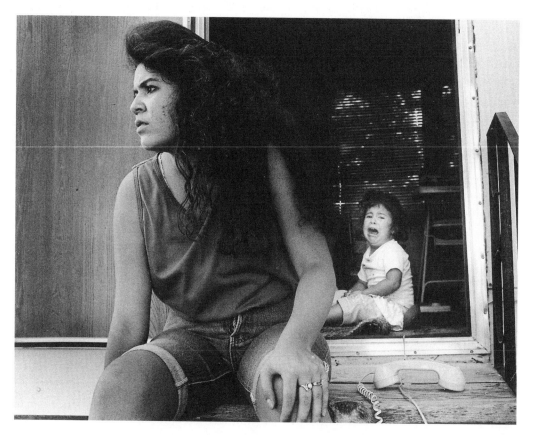

Unfortunately, examples of abuse are common. A baby continues to cry, and a frustrated teen is unable to comfort or quiet him. Eventually, the baby is hit, or shaken, and is badly injured in the process. Or a toddler is "taught" to mind her mother, for example, by being burned with a cigarette or by having her hand held over a hot stove.

"It isn't always meanness"

Social workers are quick to point out that many instances of abuse by teen parents occur not as much because of their age as because of other factors—mental illness, drug or alcohol use, or, commonly, having had parents who did the same to them. However, a great deal of the abuse is simply the result of inexperience and poor decision-making that is more common with youth.

"I had a mother come to me who had been arrested for endangerment," says one psychologist.

> She'd locked her four-month-old in a car with the windows closed on a warm day while she was inside a casino playing slot machines. I've got to tell you, she wasn't trying to punish her daughter, wasn't trying to do her harm at all. In fact, she thought she was protecting her by keeping the windows rolled up and the doors locked. It was stupidity, pure and simple. She had no idea that her child could have died.

> We need sometimes to put a monster's face on an abuser, and in many cases, that's true. But it isn't always meanness with teen parents. They just sometimes don't think like older parents would think. They aren't good at putting themselves second on the priority list, or third.[82]

And sometimes the problem is not as much abuse as it is neglect.

Not enough

Psychologists report that teen parents are more likely than older parents to neglect their children. Children who are not given the right foods or who are consistently underdressed for the weather are victims of neglect. So are babies who are never held or never played with or talked to. While neglected children do not usually bear physical scars, they do develop emotional problems that can harm them the rest of their lives.

"We see babies all too often who are emotionally neglected by young parents," says one child care worker. "The parents don't realize how important it is to interact with a very young child. I've had teenage mothers admit they let their babies cry for hours because they don't feel like getting up to change a diaper. They don't understand how babies need to feel loved, and that love comes from being held and smiled at and talked to. It's very sad."[83]

Some teen mothers realize that their own family backgrounds make it difficult to suddenly become a loving mother. One girl recognized her shortcomings and says that she's working to overcome them. "Being a mother is so hard, harder than anybody would think," she says quietly. "You have to be so patient; you have to worry all the time about someone being safe, or warm, or fed. And sometimes you just don't have the energy or the patience."[84]

4

Teen Fathers

AMERICANS AND THEIR political leaders pay a great deal of attention to teen mothers, worrying about their child-raising abilities, about the money it costs society to raise their children, and about the well-being of the children themselves. However, there is an important part of the "teens having babies" equation that is often overlooked—the teen father.

In some ways it is easy to ignore teen fathers—some counselors even label them "the invisible group." Their numbers are not defined; because they don't seek welfare benefits or financial assistance, no one really has an accurate estimate of how many teen fathers there are in the United States. Often their names don't even appear on the birth certificates of their children. In the eyes of the government agencies that assist and offer support services to teen mothers, the fathers are almost nonentities.

An unflattering stereotype

Some claim that teen fathers aren't in the picture because they don't want to be. The fact is, many young men bolt after hearing that their girlfriends are pregnant—they don't want to get entangled in a committed relationship.

Becky, a seventeen-year-old mother from Illinois, says that, for a few moments, she believed that her boyfriend was going to take responsibility for his newborn son. Immediately after the delivery, when he showed up at the hospital, Becky felt hope.

"The next day he passed out cigars to his friends," she says. "I pictured all three of us going to the zoo, doing stuff together as a family." However, she admits, his interest waned quickly. "It makes me angry that he quit coming around," Becky says. "I want to hit him."[85]

Another teen mother feels the same way. When she found out she was pregnant, her boyfriend berated her for her stupidity in not being on the pill. "He told me it wasn't no business of his, my being pregnant," she says. "And he hasn't changed his mind now that my baby is here. He's got four kids with other girls, so it ain't just me. He's got no responsibility to anybody but himself. He just looks the other way when he sees me and my baby coming."[86]

To the altar?

Many people say that teens today are less willing to take responsibility for their actions—or mistakes—than in years past. Some believe that teen parents should marry. "You married the girl, that's what you did," grumbles one man. "If you got a girl pregnant, you simply made things right and married her. Or her reputation would suffer, and yours would, too. Boys didn't think like they do now, putting themselves first and the girl second."[87]

While it is true that marriage among teen parents was far more common in years past, it is also true that, since their unwed status carries less social stigma than it might have in the past, these mothers would just as soon remain single. Many girls don't see marriage as a solution to their problems.

One girl from Boston says that marrying her boyfriend just to give her two young children a father would be far more work for her, and she's not interested in that at all. "He's a child," she says. "He whines. He expects people to do things for him. He's nasty to me. . . . He likes to sleep and watch TV. . . . The first time I met his father, who just moved up here, he asked, 'Do you want to marry him?' I looked at him and said, 'Why would I want to marry your son?' He said, 'He might grow up if you marry him.' I said, 'I can't take that chance.' No, I would not marry him. He acts like a baby and I have two of my own. I don't need him plus the kids. His mother can keep him."[88]

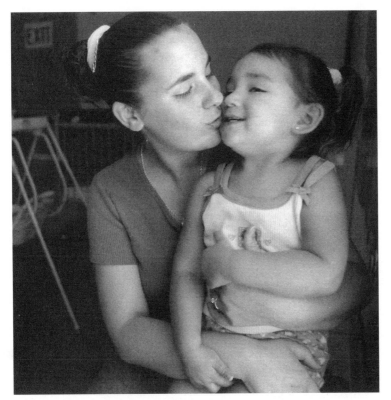

A seventeen-year-old mother made the decision to raise her two-year-old daughter on her own. Many teen mothers decide against marrying the father of their child.

"They aren't bad people"

Some experts are quick to point out that the bad behavior of many teen fathers is a function of immaturity. "They aren't bad people," says counselor Randy Brazil. "They're bad dads, yes, because most of them haven't learned what's necessary for them to become good dads. They don't have the emotional means or the financial means to make them able to understand and accept the responsibility of a child. But it certainly doesn't mean they can't learn."[89]

Teen fathers' immaturity sometimes shows itself in their denial of paternity—maintaining that the baby can't be theirs. Often a boy will accuse his girlfriend of lying about the birth control she used or of being unfaithful to him. And when all else fails, he sometimes disappears.

Jamie recalls her experience when she found out she was pregnant at fifteen. She told her boyfriend, Gary, and although she wasn't expecting marriage, she hoped he would take some responsibility for the child. Gary's reaction was disappointing. Says Jamie, "He figured that was a good time to go into the navy. So I said, 'See ya.' I guess I didn't really care, except I hated that it all turned out just like my older brothers predicted. They hated Gary, kept telling me he was never good enough for me, and then they turned out to be right."[90]

Peer pressure is a barrier

Counselors such as Randy Brazil maintain that immaturity in teen fathers can be weathered, however, just as it can be for teen mothers. "Boys need to be shown how to be good fathers," he says, "because an awful lot of them haven't had much of a role model. They lack guidance and supervision from their own fathers, and now, as a result of sexual activity, they're going to be fathers themselves. It shouldn't be a big surprise that they are tremendously unprepared."[91]

Teen fathers face severe barriers that make the step from boy to father a difficult one. One barrier is the lack of support teen fathers get from their peers. Although there is strong peer pressure to *have* sex, there is no pressure to take responsibility for the children that result from sexual activity.

"I see a lot of kids who can't wait to be considered a 'player' or a ladies' man," says one family therapist. "The whole idea of being a sexual being is so attractive to them. But it's all about taking, about keeping a tally count. It's not about listening to the other person, about really connecting on some level other than just physical. But among many teenage boys, especially lower income teens, that's the social pressure."[92]

Selective interest

And what better way to prove his sexual conquests than through impregnating girlfriends? Boys who have no clear idea of how to be supportive emotionally or financially can at least brag about the children they have fathered.

One girl recalls bitterly how the father of her little boy ignored her and the baby completely when his friends weren't around; however, when he was with his friends and saw her on the street, he'd act very interested.

Sometimes he likes to take credit for how cute Mahari looks, you know? I mean, his other kids [he has two other children with two other teen mothers] are not as cute as Mahari; in fact, they're kind of ugly. . . . So anyway, when I'm out with Mahari, and he's dressed up nice, Terry will show off for his friends. He'll be like, "Hey, look—my kid's got a new Polo hookup," or "Oh, you see my son's new Guess outfit?" Like he had anything to do with how Mahari dresses, you know? He tries to use Mahari like that.

Or he'll play this big macho thing and come up to Mahari and say, "Hey, my man" and that kind of stuff. It just scares Mahari, I think. He doesn't care about Mahari, that's for sure.[93]

Off on the wrong foot

Another barrier faced by many teen fathers is the poor relationship they have with the mother of their child. Quite often a girl discovers she is pregnant long after she has stopped seeing the father. In other cases, if a boy has not been emotionally supportive since his girlfriend gave him the news, she may withdraw from him. Knowing that he is disliked makes it difficult to summon the courage to make the first steps toward becoming a real father.

Brad, a seventeen-year-old father, says that his relationship with his girlfriend, Kim, had soured by the time she had the baby. She did not take his phone calls, and her parents would not speak to him. He knew that in the minds of Kim's parents, he had done something terrible, and they wanted him out of the picture. That made him so nervous that he was afraid to see his newborn daughter in the hospital.

I kept wondering what she looked like, if she looked anything like me. I knew from my mom [who had gone to the hospital without him] that she weighed in at 8 pounds 4 ounces when she was born, and that's pretty good-sized. I knew she had blond hair, too. I was real interested—I admit that—but I couldn't figure out a way to see the baby without getting into a scene with her parents. I was afraid.[94]

"Dead-broke dads"

One of the most formidable difficulties for teen fathers is money. By far the majority of teen fathers are completely unprepared to support—or even to help support—a baby.

"People talk about deadbeat dads," says counselor Randy Brazil, "but dead-broke dads is more like it. We're talking about a segment of the population that is either unemployed or underemployed. These are not young men who have lots of prospects, either. Many are still in high school; many have dropped out even before their girlfriends became pregnant. Without that high school diploma, without college, it's no wonder they're on the low end of the economic scale."[95]

Ironically, however, it is money that seems to be the demand made of teen fathers. More and more states are making blood testing mandatory so that a child's true paternity can be established. In these states, once the tests prove who

A teen father holds his daughter. Teen fathers are expected to support their kids financially, but often do not have the means to do so.

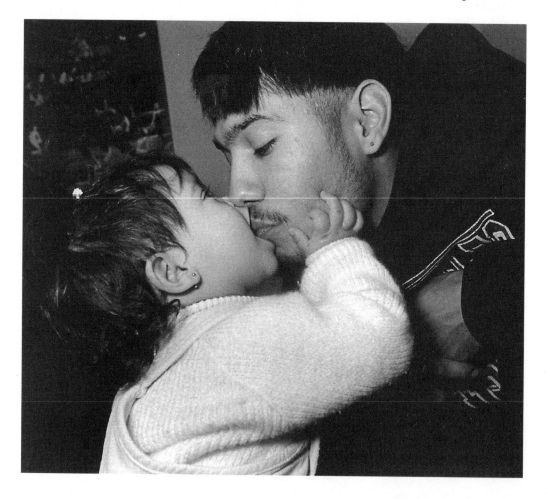

the father is, he can be held accountable financially for child support. In fact, he can even lose his driver's license or have his wages garnished if he fails to pay up.

Harder than it used to be

The financial situation for a teen father is far grimmer than it was in times past. In the 1960s and 1970s, for example, a teenage boy had a far easier time supporting a wife (marriage was the usual result of an unplanned teen pregnancy then) and child. Because of the abundance of jobs that paid well and required little training, there were far more opportunities for teenagers to earn the money they needed.

"I had my first daughter when I was seventeen," remembers one Chicago auto dealer.

> It was 1964, and believe it or not, it wasn't as big a deal as it would be for me now! I was working part-time for my uncle's garage. I was earning good money, too. So when Moira told me she was pregnant, I dropped out of my senior year of high school and got on at my uncle's full-time.

> Nowadays, I know how hard that would be. First of all, most of the jobs teenagers can get now are flipping burgers at McDonald's, or carrying grocery bags at the supermarket. They probably get minimum wage, and that's not enough for even the kid himself to live on![96]

Statistics today certainly support the perception that teen fathers are in a precarious position. In the twenty years between 1973 and 1993, for instance, the median weekly earnings of young men sixteen to twenty-four working full-time fell almost 30 percent. (Older males made less money, too, but their earnings fell by only 7 percent in the same period.) Although a number of factors are to blame for the decrease in earnings, economists say the main reason is the decrease in the number of jobs that don't require specialized training coupled with the increase in the number of minimum-wage jobs.

The few low-skill, high-pay jobs that remain are hard to get. "There's a great deal of competition out there for such jobs," a high school vocational counselor explains. "While a young man who could do auto repair or plumbing could

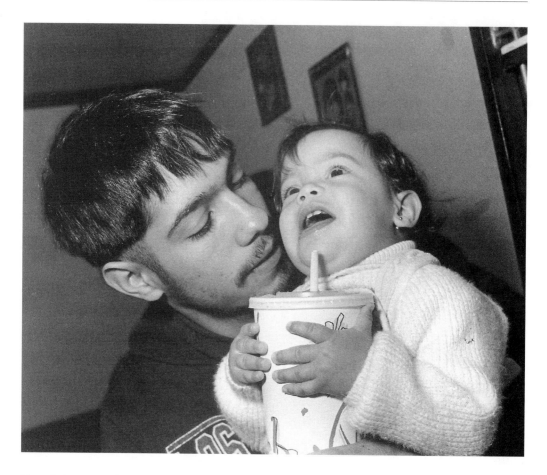

Teen fathers can play an important and valuable role in their child's life without providing financial support.

easily find work thirty years ago, today these same jobs are extremely hard to find—and even then, they require licensing or trade school."[97]

More than just a paycheck

But finances—or lack of them—should not stand in the way of teen fathers' getting involved with their children, say experts. There are valuable aspects of being a father that have nothing whatsoever to do with money.

"It's a complete myth that outside of a paycheck, teen fathers have nothing to offer," says Randy Brazil. "Social workers and counselors are starting to see that now. We know of lots of ways that teens can bring something very positive to their children. They aren't 'throwaway dads,' as they were once called."[98]

Forming bonds with a young child lays the foundation for that child to have good relationships with adults in the future. By watching a father in day-to-day dealings with other people, a child gradually understands courtesy and respect. For qualities such as honesty and patience, a father is an excellent role model.

"There's no arguing it," says one counselor. "A father's presence in the home is a stabilizing factor. Mothers—no matter how much child support they receive—cannot and should not do it alone."[99]

But how?

There are a number of ways that teen fathers can get involved in their children's lives; however, many need help understanding how to begin. This is why some communities are taking steps to ensure that young fathers can learn how to be supportive—not only financially but emotionally and developmentally.

One program that has achieved a great deal of success is Minnesota Early Learning Design (MELD) for Young Dads, which has spread from Minneapolis to many other cities in the United States. Classes at MELD educate young fathers on a number of topics, ranging from birth control options to finding and keeping jobs that would support their new families to the correct way to bathe and diaper an infant.

The classes are taught by men who were teen fathers themselves; this means that the teachers can relate to what the fathers are feeling or to questions that they might have. Few of those attending the classes have the necessary skills to do much of anything at first, but they learn quickly.

"I have young men of sixteen, seventeen, who are so afraid of the baby's size, about doing anything that might hurt their baby, they're almost terrified to pick it up," says one teacher. "They're scared that the baby's crying means that they're doing something wrong. It's a relief for them to learn that sometimes babies just cry, that a father can be just a guy who holds the baby, walks with it until it falls asleep."[100]

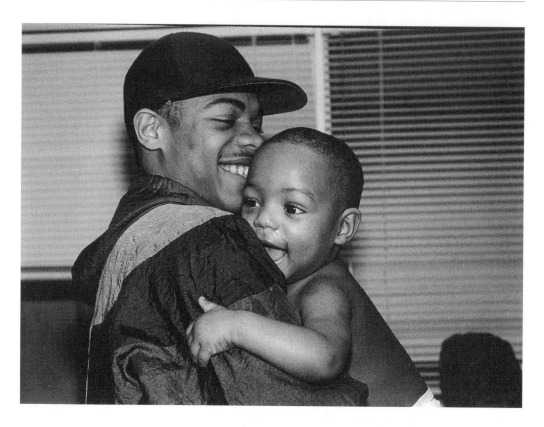

More teen fathers are learning how to be good parents through community education programs.

They don't know how important they are

What is interesting to many men who staff teen parent resource centers is that more than 80 percent of the teen fathers they see have no relationship with their own fathers. Many of them are surprised to realize the importance of a father in a child's life.

"If he hasn't ever really known his father, he doesn't know what a big deal it is," says one teacher. "That sixteen-year-old boy with a little baby may feel totally out of his element now. But you know why we need to start on that boy now? Because in ten years, he's going to be twenty-six, and the father of a ten-year-old. And by then, if the father hasn't gotten involved in some way, that ten-year-old will be just another kid in a fragile family structure who has grown up without a father."

"It takes commitment, it takes a will," he continues. "And it's hard, because you're taking a teenager, who only thinks of himself—that's where he is developmentally—and get him to focus on someone else. Making sure that baby is fed, is warm, is safe. It's a hard job, but these teen fathers can do it. I've seen it happen. And the thing most of these dads say to me is, 'I don't want to be the kind of father I had. I want to be there for my son, or my daughter, because my father was never there for me.'"[101]

5

What Can Be Done?

WITH SO MANY babies being born to teenagers each year, and with the dire consequences predicted for those children's well-being, it is not surprising that there are many people who consider the issue of teen parenting an urgent one. It is also not surprising that there are often conflicting ideas about what programs or solutions are best.

One of the most critical aspects of being a teen parent is the lack of money. The majority of teen mothers are finding it almost impossible to climb above poverty level. Teen fathers who admit paternity and wish to help out are usually in no better shape financially than the mothers themselves. How can teen parents and their children survive?

The welfare system

Welfare is the most common financial crutch today for teen parents and their children. Assistance programs at the county, state, and federal levels provide teen parents and their children with food stamps, free infant formula, reduced child care and housing, and cash.

The federal welfare system was developed in the 1930s during the Great Depression. The primary intent was to provide help to families in which the "breadwinner" (most often the husband) had died or had just deserted his wife and children. The typical welfare recipient was therefore a widowed or deserted woman. The expectation was that she would be on welfare only until she could find another means of supporting her family. The modern welfare recipient is different: She is more often a woman who is divorced, is separated, or has never been married.

Public sympathy erodes

Teenage mothers form the core of the welfare population, consuming more than $34 billion in benefits each year. And while the original idea of welfare was to provide assistance temporarily until the family could get back on its feet, these teen mothers are the segment of the population that is least likely to escape poverty.

Many people feel that the government should not be supplying aid to young people having babies out of wedlock. They argue that giving out such benefits to people with such poor prospects for the future is simply adding to the problem.

"A lot of people are asking whether instead of helping mothers raise their children, the government isn't contributing to a breakdown in the family," says Lila Jeffries, a

A single mom seeks help at a homeless shelter. Under new federal laws, teens who don't live at home face the loss of welfare benefits.

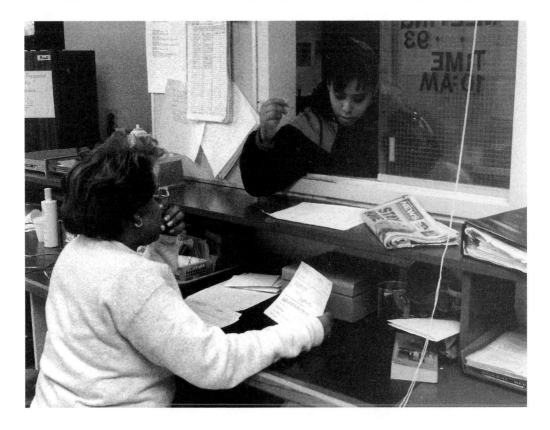

social service worker from Minneapolis. "So many single-parent families, so many babies being born out of wedlock. And it's the mothers who are blamed, I guess. The term *welfare mother* has become a slur in our society."[102]

An enticement?

Some criticism has gone even farther than moral outrage against unmarried mothers. Many people have charged that by providing money for each child, the welfare system is actually encouraging teens to have babies. Rather than providing a temporary safety net, they maintain, over the years welfare has become an enticing trap.

Robert Rector, in his 1995 study "America's Failed $5.4 Trillion War on Poverty," claims the program is highly suspect and damaging not only to recipients of welfare but also to the American taxpayer. "In welfare, as in most other things," he writes, "you get what you pay for—and for 30 years the welfare system has paid for non-work and non-marriage. Now we have massive increases in both, and an explosion of illegitimacy, which breeds all manner of social ills. . . . By undermining the work ethic and rewarding illegitimacy, the welfare system thus insidiously generates its own clientele."[103]

At least in part as an answer to such criticism, Congress passed a welfare reform bill in August 1996. The legislation, subsequently signed by President Bill Clinton, contained provisions that lawmakers hoped would reduce the number of teen parents. The law stated that teen mothers who wish to receive federal welfare benefits must comply with two stipulations: They must live at home and they must continue to go to school. Noncompliance with either of these rules would mean a loss of benefits.

More legislation followed. By 1997 new federal laws limited the time that a woman may remain on the welfare rolls. Going even beyond the federal guidelines, many states have enacted their own limitations for assistance, such as cutting off benefits for women—many of whom are teen mothers—who continue to have children while on welfare. The idea, said government officials, was to send a clear message that the "safety net" was meant to be temporary, not a way of life.

Surprising critics

It isn't just fiscal or political conservatives who find fault with the welfare system. Teen mothers are some of the harshest critics of welfare—a fact that surprises some people. Kari, seventeen, says that anyone who thinks welfare benefits bring with them an easy way of life is kidding themselves.

> I get WIC [Women, Infants, and Children] for free formula and some housing help. I get $260 each month in food stamps. But that means I don't save a dime. I'm living in a bad neighborhood, and I'm trying to get enough money to move. I'm within like three or four dollars of my budget every month. Somebody in Washington or whatever says I'm a welfare queen? Yeah, right.
>
> I say if you are going to make welfare like that, then why bother? I want to work. But if I work, I get no benefits, and right now, the benefits are more than work would be at the mall or wherever. I'm going back to school when there's a space at the day care for my baby. We're on a waiting list. But until I got me that diploma or whatever, I'm stuck.[104]

Others argue that the system not only makes it financially harder to work, but it discourages fathers from becoming involved in the raising of their children. One social worker recalls a woman he recently counseled who had what is considered an average packet of benefits for a single mother of two small children:

> She was getting about $280 per month in AFDC, $300 per month [in] food stamps, Medicaid (no amount mentioned, but call it at least $100 a month—certainly the insurance for a woman and two kids would be that much), and she was about to get housing (say, $350 a month in Houston). This doesn't even count all the other little [benefits] that she can get as long as she's a single parent—fuel assistance, free job training, day care during the job training, supplemental social security—that all disappears if she marries. (Well, she might get to keep some of the food stamps and some of the AFDC, depending on his income. But she loses the housing, even if he's unemployed.)[105]

Helping teen parents stay in school

Though many teen parents realize that an education is the only way out of the cycle of poverty and welfare, staying in school can be a daunting task. Teen fathers who try to become involved by contributing financially to their children's upkeep may need to drop out of school in order to keep a full-time (though usually low-paying) job.

For teen mothers—usually the full-time caregivers of their children—attending school is almost too difficult to imagine. "How could I do that," wonders one teen mother, "when I'm busy all day with my little boy? My boyfriend comes around like once a week, and he's working. My mama's working, and who am I supposed to pay to watch my son while I'm writing book reports or something? And with what money?"[106]

To make education a more attainable goal, many high schools have begun on-site day care for teen parents. For a moderate fee (anywhere from $1 to $6 daily) a teen can drop off the child and attend classes. In addition to saving money and time by eliminating extra trips to day care centers, the parent has the peace of mind that the child is very close by.

One seventeen-year-old mother who attends high school in Reading, Pennsylvania, says that she is grateful that her school offers day care, for it enables her to spend some time during her school day with her three-month-old daughter. "Every day I come down during lunch," she says. "Usually when I come down, she's crying, so I just go in there and play with her to get her relaxed. Then I come out here and eat and then go back in."[107]

A silver platter?

Many teens who use high school day care centers admit that without such a convenience, they would have dropped out of school. Although there are some who feel that, by helping teen parents in this way, the community is giving its approval to their life choices, the alternative to such help seems just as bad. "The first impression is that we're handing these girls everything on a silver platter," says the coordinator of one center. "But what's the alternative? Out of school, pregnant, and on welfare?"[108]

Indeed, many conservative lawmakers feel that making teen parenting as difficult and uncomfortable as possible is the best way to discourage teens from having babies in the first place. One congressional staff member who supports cuts in welfare benefits complains, "The federal government has made it possible through welfare for unwed women to have babies without having to suffer."[109] And if young mothers do "suffer," or at least are inconvenienced, some critics of the centers believe that teens will be discouraged from having babies they cannot adequately support.

Two teen mothers take their children to a day care center at a high school in Minneapolis. Many conservative politicians disapprove of such publicly funded centers, seeing them as enticements for teens to have children.

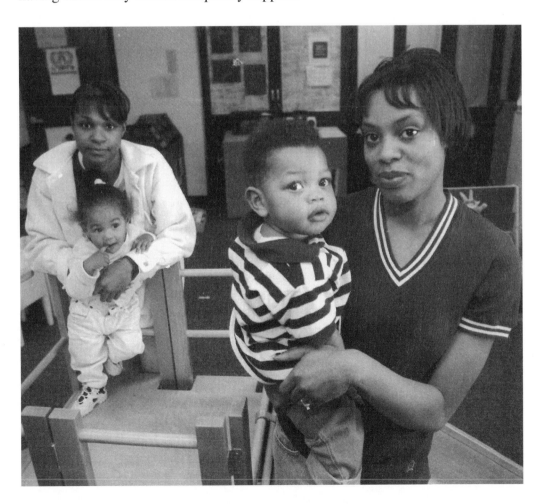

However, there are many who feel that cutting benefits to teenage mothers and their children will only create more problems. They point to the rapidly growing numbers of homeless families who are in need of shelter, food, and medical care. They predict that by taking benefits away from teen parents we will be adding to those numbers.

"What this society *does not* need," says one shelter worker firmly, "is more homeless people. But you take money and educational opportunities from these young moms, and how do we expect them to survive? I see too many of them now at our center, fourteen- and fifteen-year-old girls with babies. Most have no home to go back to; many left because of abuse. God, it makes me so mad to hear these politicians talk about punishing these young moms. It's like we think they're living it up at the taxpayers' expense! I can see being frustrated at the stupid decisions many teenagers make, but why punish their babies?"[110]

Maternity homes

Instead of wanting to eliminate welfare entirely, some politicians and those who work with teens endorse the idea of requiring teen mothers to live in group homes as a condition of receiving welfare benefits. Some suggest that unmarried pregnant teens, who normally would receive cash and other benefits from AFDC and other programs, are better off living away from home. Too often, say counselors, they have no supervision from their own parents and, as a result, can slide into a lifestyle that is hazardous to their unborn babies as well as to themselves.

"Home is often the source of the problems," says one social worker. "The lack of supervision, the lack of parent involvement resulted in the pregnancy in the first place. A lot of the girls we see come from homes where drugs and alcohol are prevalent, and where family violence is a way of life."[111]

The answer, say many, is to establish dormitory-style residences where health care workers and adolescent counselors can supervise teens during their pregnancy as well as during the early part of their motherhood. There they can get the information they need to become good mothers and at the same time devote time to finishing high school.

However, some are critical of the maternity home idea. They say that whatever bad influences exist in the teen's home and neighborhood cannot be avoided simply by moving. "Do they really believe the prospect of living in group homes with other unwed mothers will counteract the influence of peer pressure, which is pushing kids into sexual activity at younger and younger ages?" wonders one critic. "Have any of them ever watched 'Beverly Hills 90210' . . . or any of the shows aimed at adolescents in which sexual activity among the young is neither shameful or surprising?"[112]

Other critics say that the plan would be expensive and that the money it would take to feed, clothe, educate, and otherwise monitor teen mothers and their babies could be better spent on programs aimed at preventing pregnancy.

Sex education

Many people involved in the counseling of teen parents say that the best answer is to prevent teens from becoming parents in the first place through improved education. Welfare programs, teen father resources, and even group homes may ease the plight of teen parents, but the real answer is to somehow stop the need for such things to begin with. President Clinton in one budget request allotted $400 million for sex education in schools located in poor urban neighborhoods. There are very different ideas, however, about what kind of curriculum is most effective.

Some say that since teens are almost sure to engage in sexual activity, sex education should concentrate on methods of contraception and minimizing the risk of sexually transmitted diseases (STDs). As writers for the Alan Guttmacher Institute state in their family planning policy statement, "If adults are going to help teenagers avoid the outcomes of sex that are clearly negative—STDs, unintended pregnancies, abortions, and out-of-wedlock births—they must accept the

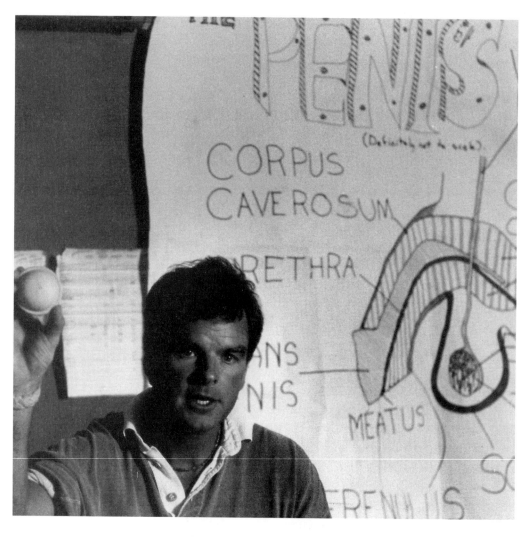

Sex education is looked upon as one of the best means of preventing teen pregnancies. Controversy exists however, over how these classes should be taught.

reality of adolescent sexual activity and deal with it directly and honestly."[113]

However, there are strong arguments against this type of curriculum. No contraceptive method is 100 percent effective, and to teach teens to rely on birth control alone to avoid pregnancy is a limited answer. For example, even Planned Parenthood—an organization widely known for supporting sex education—showed in 1993 that condoms, the most common method of contraception used by teens, have a 15.7 percent failure rate at preventing pregnancy over the course of a year.

The reverse effect?

Furthermore, some believe that teaching the use of contraception and providing increased access to condoms and other methods of birth control encourage more sexual activity among teens without encouraging responsible behavior. Chicago's Cardinal Bernadin spoke for many Catholics when he doubted whether "more and better contraceptive information and services will make major inroads in the number of teenage pregnancies—it will motivate them to precocious sexual activity but by no means to the practice of contraception."[114]

Rather than accepting the idea that teens will have sex, some say, it is far better to encourage abstinence among teenagers by stressing the consequences of such activity. Knowing that the logical outcome of sexual activity is a baby, many teens might rethink their views on sex. While some scoff at the notion that teens would take the idea of abstinence seriously, some teens say that, whether because

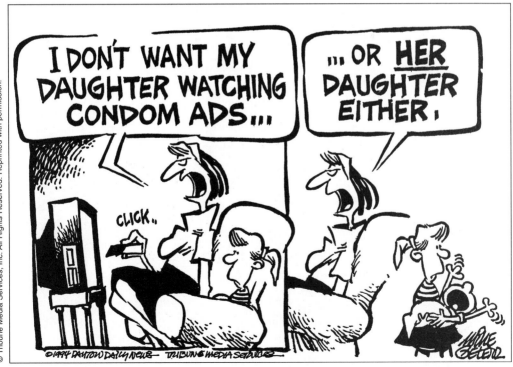

of abstinence discussions in school sex education programs or because of their own belief systems, they have chosen abstinence at this point in their lives.

"I know that if I were to have sex and get a girl pregnant, I wouldn't run away," says an eighteen-year-old North Carolina football player. "I wouldn't be able to go to college. I'd need to stay here and help take care of the baby. And with a kid, it's going to be twenty-four hours a day—constantly—for eighteen years."[115]

Another teen, fifteen-year-old Denise, says that she and her boyfriend have decided to put off sexual activity indefinitely. "I don't want to commit something like that without being married, or at least being sure I'm in love," she says. "I've heard so many sad stories about people who just do it for the sake of doing it and feeling bad about it later. I don't want that to be me—sex has to be more special than that."[116]

"I wish I'd never had this baby"

Some of the most plaintive voices are those of teen parents themselves. They have experienced the difficulties of an unplanned pregnancy and the financial and emotional uncertainty that accompanies it.

Kara, sixteen, says she loves her son but she wishes she'd never gotten pregnant. "I wouldn't harm a hair on his head," she says, crying. "But I wish I'd never had him, I wish I'd never had this baby. I don't know if I'll ever have a normal life, and I know motherhood is good for some people, but I'm not ready yet."[117]

Many teens say that they feel cheated, that they missed out on a part of life that they can never recover. Jamie, a twenty-five-year-old mother who gave birth to her oldest child when she was in ninth grade, admits that she's had more than a few regrets. "When I was pregnant with Richard, I went down to Memphis to see my cousin graduate from high school," she remembers. "While I was there, I helped her get ready for her senior prom. The whole time I'm thinking, 'Yeah, I've got my babies, and I'm glad.' But there was another part of me that was thinking, 'You'll never know what it feels like to go to the prom either.'"[118]

While teen parents may experience varying degrees of success in different aspects of their lives, most would agree that to be a good and nurturing parent at any age is a challenge. But to be that parent as a teenager is inarguably the most difficult long-term occupation any could imagine.

Notes

Introduction

1. Interview with the author, Minneapolis, MN, May 1995.

2. Interview with the author, Minneapolis, MN, July 1995.

3. Interview with the author, Minneapolis, MN, July 1995.

4. Rebecca A. Maynard, ed., *Kids Having Kids: Economic Costs and Social Consequences of Teen Pregnancy.* Washington, DC: Urban Institute Press, 1997, p. 1.

5. Quoted in Janet Bode, *Kids Still Having Kids: People Talk About Teen Pregnancy.* New York: Franklin Watts, 1992, p. 60.

6. Interview with the author, Minneapolis, MN, August 1999.

7. Quoted in Joelle Sander, *Before Their Time: Four Generations of Teenage Mothers.* New York: Harcourt Brace Jovanovich, 1991, p. 40.

8. Kristin Luker, *Dubious Conceptions: The Politics of Teenage Pregnancy.* Cambridge, MA: Harvard University Press, 1996, p. 2.

9. Quoted in Sander, *Before Their Time,* p. 40.

10. Quoted in Sander, *Before Their Time,* p. 72.

11. Interview with the author, Minneapolis, MN, March 1997.

Chapter 1: The Increase in Teen Pregnancy

12. Interview with the author, Minneapolis, MN, July 1999.

13. Interview with the author, Minneapolis, MN, July 1995.

14. Interview with the author, St. Paul, MN, May 1995.

15. Quoted in Terri Peterson Smith, "Up Close at a Distance: Staying Involved in Your Adolescent's Education," *Better Homes and Gardens,* September 1996, p. 220.

16. Interview with the author, Minneapolis, MN, March 1997.

17. Interview with the author, Minneapolis, MN, September 1999.

18. Ron Stodghill, "Where'd You Learn That?" *Time,* June 15, 1998, p. 57.

19. Quoted in Stodghill, "Where'd You Learn That?" p. 58.

20. Quoted in Luker, *Dubious Conceptions,* p. 140.

21. Quoted in Stodghill, "Where'd You Learn That?" p. 57.

22. Quoted in Stodghill, "Where'd You Learn That?" p. 55.

23. Quoted in Gracie Bonds Staples, "Teen Pregnancy Exacts a High Price from All of Us," *Fort Worth Star-Telegram,* June 1, 1999, p. K7.

24. Quoted in Bode, *Kids Still Having Kids,* p. 18.

25. Interview with the author, Minneapolis, MN, June 1995.

26. Quoted in Jan Farrington, "Sex and Responsibility: What Does the 'R' Word Mean to You?" *Current Health 2,* September 1995, p. 3.

27. Quoted in Elizabeth Karlsberg, "How Far Would You Go to Fit In?" *Teen Magazine,* January 1996, p. 53.

28. Quoted in Luker, *Dubious Conceptions,* p. 141.

29. Quoted in Luker, *Dubious Conceptions,* p. 139.

30. Interview with the author, Minneapolis, MN, May 1995.

31. Interview with the author, Minneapolis, MN, April 1995.

32. Quoted in Bode, *Kids Still Having Kids,* p. 87.

33. Interview with the author, Minneapolis, MN, July 1995.

34. Quoted in Bode, *Kids Still Having Kids,* pp. 18–19.

35. Interview with the author, Minneapolis, MN, March 1997.

36. Quoted in Allison Bell, "Pregnant on Purpose," *Teen Magazine,* August 1997, p. 107.

37. Interview with the author, Minneapolis, MN, July 1995.

38. Interview with the author, Minneapolis, MN, July 1995.

39. Quoted in Bell, "Pregnant on Purpose," p. 106.

40. Interview with the author, Minneapolis, MN, July 1995.

41. Quoted in Luker, Dubious Conceptions, p. 151.

Chapter 2: "What Do I Do Now?"

42. Interview with the author, Minneapolis, MN, June 1995.

43. Quoted in Bode, *Kids Still Having Kids,* p. 85.

44. Interview with the author, Minneapolis, MN, March 1997.

45. Interview with the author, Minneapolis, MN, June 1995.

46. Interview with the author, Minneapolis, MN, August 1995.

47. Interview with the author, Minneapolis, MN, August 1995.

48. Interview with the author, Minneapolis, MN, June 1995.

49. Interview with the author, Minneapolis, MN, May 1996.

50. Interview with the author, Minneapolis, MN, May 1995.

51. Interview with the author, Minneapolis, MN, June 1995.

52. Interview with the author, Minneapolis, MN, May 1995.

53. Interview with the author, Minneapolis, MN, June 1998.

54. Interview with the author, Minneapolis, MN, July 1995.

55. Interview with the author, Minneapolis, MN, June 1995.

56. Luker, *Dubious Conceptions,* p. 162.

57. Quoted in Luker, *Dubious Conceptions*, p. 163.

58. Interview with the author, Minneapolis, MN, July 1995.

59. Quoted in Stephen P. Thompson, ed., *Teenage Pregnancy: Opposing Viewpoints.* San Diego: Greenhaven Press, 1997, p. 70.

60. Interview with the author, Minneapolis, MN, July 1995.

61. Interview with the author, Minneapolis, MN, June 1995.

Chapter 3: The Challenges of Parenthood

62. Interview with the author, Minneapolis, MN, August 1995.

63. Interview with the author, Minneapolis, MN, August 1995.

64. Interview with the author, Minneapolis, MN, July 1995.

65. Interview with the author, Minneapolis, MN, June 1995.

66. Interview with the author, Minneapolis, MN, August 1995.

67. Interview with the author, Minneapolis, MN, May 1995.

68. Interview with the author, Minneapolis, MN, August 1995.

69. Interview with the author, Minneapolis, MN, August 1999.

70. Interview with the author, Bloomington, MN, July 1999.

71. Interview with the author, St. Paul, MN, August 1995.

72. Interview with the author, St. Paul, MN, August 1995.

73. Interview with the author, Minneapolis, MN, August 1995.

74. Interview with the author, Minneapolis, MN, August 1995.

75. Interview with the author, Minneapolis, MN, August 1995.

76. Interview with the author, Minneapolis, MN, March 1997.

77. Interview with the author, Minneapolis, MN, August 1999.

78. Interview with the author, St. Paul, MN, April 1997.

79. Interview with the author, Minneapolis, MN, May 1997.

80. Interview with the author, Minneapolis, MN, August 1995.

81. Interview with the author, Minneapolis, MN, August 1999.

82. Interview with the author, Minneapolis, MN, March 1996.

83. Interview with the author, Minneapolis, MN, August 1999.

84. Interview with the author, Minneapolis, MN, July 1996.

Chapter 4: Teen Fathers

85. Quoted in "Reality Bites," *People Weekly,* November 27, 1995, p. 53.

86. Interview with the author, Minneapolis, MN, June 1995.

87. Interview with the author, Minneapolis, MN, August 1999.

88. Quoted in Luker, *Dubious Conceptions,* p. 159.

89. Interview with the author, Minneapolis, MN, August 1999.

90. Interview with the author, Rogers, MN, March 1998.

91. Interview with the author, Minneapolis, MN, August 1999.

92. Interview with the author, Minneapolis, MN, August 1999.

93. Interview with the author, Minneapolis, MN, July 1995.

94. Interview with the author, Minneapolis, MN, March 1997.

95. Interview with the author, Minneapolis, MN, August 1999.

96. Interview with the author, Minneapolis, MN, March 1997.

97. Interview with the author, Minneapolis, MN, March 1997.

98. Interview with the author, Minneapolis, MN, August 1999.

99. Interview with the author, Minneapolis, MN, July 1995.

100. Interview with the author, Minneapolis, MN, July 1995.

101. Interview with the author, Minneapolis, MN, August 1999.

Chapter 5: What Can Be Done?

102. Interview with the author, St. Paul, MN, January 1997.

103. Quoted in Thompson, *Teenage Pregnancy,* p. 65.

104. Interview with the author, Minneapolis, MN, January 1997.

105. Quoted in Gail Stewart, *Teen Fathers: The Other America.* San Diego: Lucent Books, 1998, p. 11.

106. Interview with the author, Minneapolis, MN, March 1997.

107. Quoted in "Book Bags and Baby Bottles," *Scholastic Update,* March 10, 1995, p. 129.

108. Quoted in "Book Bags and Baby Bottles," p. 128.

109. Quoted in Thompson, *Teenage Pregnancy,* pp. 13–14.

110. Interview with the author, Minneapolis, MN, August 1995.

111. Interview with the author, Minneapolis, MN, September 1999.

112. Quoted in Thompson, *Teenage Pregnancy,* p. 152.

113. Alan Guttmacher Institute, *Sex and America's Teenagers.* New York: Alan Guttmacher Institute, 1994.

114. Quoted in Thompson, *Teenage Pregnancy,* p. 96.

115. Quoted in Gayle Forman, "Sex? No Thanks! Four Guy Virgins Tell Why They're Waiting," *Seventeen,* August 1999, p. 257.

116. Interview with the author, Minneapolis, MN, August 1999.

117. Interview with the author, Minneapolis, MN, August 1995.

118. Interview with the author, Minneapolis, MN, March 1997.

Organizations
to Contact

The following organizations can be contacted for more information about teen parenting.

The Alan Guttmacher Institute
120 Wall St.
New York, NY 10005
e-mail: info@agi-usa.org

This organization works to help men and women have access to information and services necessary to exercise their rights and responsibilities concerning sexual activities, reproduction, and family planning.

National Organization of Adolescent Pregnancy, Parenting, and Prevention
1319 F St. NW, Suite 401
Washington, DC 20004
e-mail: noapp@aol.com

This organization supports families in setting standards that encourage the healthy development of children in loving, stable relationships. It works for the prevention and resolution of problems associated with teen pregnancy and parenthood.

Project Reality
P.O. Box 97
Golf, IL 60029

This organization encourages abstinence as the best pregnancy preventative, and has developed an educational curriculum for junior and senior high school students.

Sex Information and Education Council of the U.S.
130 W. 42nd St., Suite 2500
New York, NY 10036

This is one of the largest clearinghouses for information about pregnancy and related issues.

Suggestions for Further Reading

Shirley Arthur, *Surviving Teen Pregnancy: Your Choices, Dreams, and Decisions.* Buena Park, CA: Morning Glory Press, 1996. Very readable, with an excellent bibliography.

Robert Coles, *The Youngest Parents.* New York: Double Take Books, 1997. Well written; contains wonderful photographs to illustrate the lives of the people interviewed.

Jeanne Warren Lindsay, *Teen Dads: Rights, Responsibilities and Joys.* Buena Park, CA: Morning Glory Press, 1993. Although written for an audience of teen fathers or fathers-to-be, this book has a very well written section on problems of getting along with the baby's mother.

Gail Stewart, *Teen Fathers: The Other America.* San Diego: Lucent Books, 1998. First-person accounts by a varied group of teen fathers.

Periodicals

"Book Bags and Baby Bottles," *Scholastic Update,* March 10, 1995.

Gayle Forman, "Sex? No Thanks! Four Guy Virgins Tell Why They're Waiting," *Seventeen,* August 1999.

Donald Lambro, "Welfare Increases Poverty and Illegitimacy," *Conservative Chronicle,* June 28, 1995.

Works Consulted

Alan Guttmacher Institute, *Sex and America's Teenagers.* New York: Alan Guttmacher Institute, 1994. Good information on contraceptive use among teens.

Janet Bode, *Kids Still Having Kids: People Talk About Teen Pregnancy.* New York: Franklin Watts, 1992. Very readable accounts from teen parents, doctors, and counselors.

Kristin Luker, *Dubious Conceptions: The Politics of Teenage Pregnancy.* Cambridge, MA: Harvard University Press, 1996. Good background material on the historical aspect of teen parenting; helpful chapter on why pregnant teens choose to raise their own children.

Rebecca A. Maynard, ed., *Kids Having Kids: Economic Costs and Social Consequences of Teen Pregnancy.* Washington, DC: Urban Institute Press, 1997. Difficult reading but very pertinent statistical information, especially regarding child abuse and teen parents.

Joelle Sander, *Before Their Time: Four Generations of Teenage Mothers.* New York: Harcourt Brace Jovanovich, 1991. Excellent interviews, with good information on teen mothers during the years of World War II.

Stephen P. Thompson, ed., *Teenage Pregnancy: Opposing Viewpoints.* San Diego: Greenhaven Press, 1997. Excellent background material on welfare; helpful introduction.

Periodicals

Allison Bell, "Pregnant on Purpose," *Teen Magazine,* August 1997.

Janet Coburn, "Child Care in High Schools," *School Planning and Management,* January 1999.

Kristi Collier, "Pregnant . . . Now What?" *Teen Magazine,* April 1996.

Jan Farrington, "Sex and Responsibility: What Does the 'R' Word Mean to You?" *Current Health 2,* September 1995.

Elizabeth Karlsberg, "How Far Would You Go to Fit In?" *Teen Magazine,* January 1996.

Jane Mauldon and Kristin Luker, "Does Liberalism Cause Sex?" *American Prospect,* Winter 1996.

"Reality Bites," *People Weekly,* November 27, 1995.

Terri Peterson Smith, "Up Close at a Distance: Staying Involved in Your Adolescent's Education," *Better Homes and Gardens,* September 1996.

Gracie Bonds Staples, "Teen Pregnancy Exacts a High Price from All of Us," *Fort Worth Star-Telegram,* June 1, 1999.

Ron Stodghill, "Where'd You Learn That?" *Time,* June 15, 1998.

"Teaching Teen Mothers," *U.S. Catholic,* May 1995.

Index

Picture Credits

About the Author

Gail B. Stewart received her undergraduate degree from Gustavus Adolphus College in St. Peter, Minnesota. She did her graduate work in English, linguistics, and curriculum study at the College of St. Thomas and the University of Minnesota. She taught English and reading for more than ten years.

She has written over ninety books for young people, including a series for Lucent Books called *The Other America*. She has written many books on historical topics such as World War I and the Warsaw Ghetto.

Stewart and her husband live in Minneapolis with their three sons, Ted, Elliot, and Flynn, two dogs, and a cat. When she is not writing she enjoys reading, walking, and watching her sons play soccer.